GETTING OFF THE

PAIN

ROLLER

COASTER

Psychological Aspects of Pain
and Pain Management

Barry W. Weiss, Ph. D.

Lillie Weiss, Ph.D.

Other Books by Lillie Weiss:

Treating Bulimia
You Can't Have Your Cake and Eat It Too
Dream Analysis in Psychotherapy
Women's Conflicts About Eating and Sexuality
    (also published as *Good Girls Don't Eat Dessert)*

Library of Congress Cataloging-in-Publication Data
Weiss, Barry W.
    Getting Off the Pain Roller Coaster: Psychological Aspects of Pain
    and Pain Management / Barry W. Weiss, Lillie Weiss ; drawings by
    Yvonne Arnett ; graphics by Mary Kay Childs.
        p.   cm.
    Includes bibliographical references.
    ISBN # 0-9645528-0-9
    1. Pain—Psychological aspects.   2. Pain—Treatment.
    I. Weiss, Lillie.   II. Title
    [DNLM: 1. Pain—prevention & control.   2. Pain—psychology.
    WL 704 W429g 1994]
RB 127.W45   1994
616'.0472—dc20
DNLM/DLC
for Library of Congress   95-7614
                                                              CIP

Printed in the United States of America

Information in this book is deemed to be authentic and accurate by
authors and publisher. However, they disclaim any liability incurred
in connection with the use of information appearing in this book.

Golden Psych Press
Phoenix, Arizona

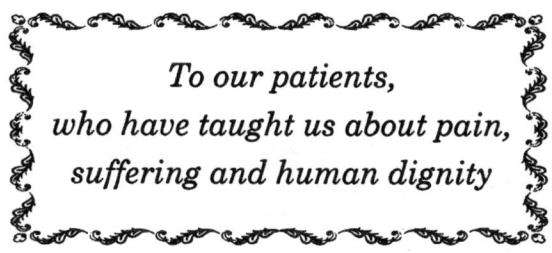

To our patients,
who have taught us about pain,
suffering and human dignity

Acknowledgments

The birth of a book is not unlike the birth of a child, and we would like to thank the many people who have helped us in this birth process. Our patients, to whom this book is dedicated, have of course provided us with the material, and we are grateful to Lou and others for sharing their stories with us.

Our thanks goes to the staff at The Book Studio who have ensured a smooth, safe and unusually speedy delivery. We thank them for their professionalism and for going above and beyond the necessary. They have exemplified quality, service and pride in their work. We are grateful to them for all of their input and for their many helpful suggestions which have contributed so much to the overall presentation and quality of the final production.

We would also like to thank Mary Kay for her skillful typing of the manuscript — over and over! — and for her cheerful meeting of deadlines. We are indebted to her for her innovative treatment of our concepts and for her creative ideas which have enhanced the appearance of this book.

We are also grateful to Yvonne for translating our ideas into artistic and humorous creations which have contributed so much to the overall quality of this book.

Most births are accompanied by labor pains, and this one was no exception. Last but not least, we are indebted to Robin for helping us get off our own pain roller coaster in severing the cord that was strangling this baby.

Table of Contents

Preface

Life with chronic pain can seem like an emotional roller coaster ride. We wrote this book for anyone who has lived with pain longer than necessary, for anyone who has had to limit his or her activities because of the pain, for anyone who has ever questioned his or her meaning in life because of these limitations—and for their families, friends, employers and members of the health care profession who deal with them. It is for those who want to learn to control their pain rather than let it control them.

Pain is a condition that disrupts the lives of millions of people daily—the people who suffer from it, their loved ones, their employers and their health providers. It is estimated that one in five Americans suffers from chronic pain—pain which lasts longer than six months. Millions of people hear these words from their doctors: "There is nothing more I can do for you—you just have to learn to live with the pain." Many see it as a death sentence when they hear they may never work again or do the things they enjoyed before.

Pain is a crisis that hits at the very core of one's being and pervades every aspect of one's life—family, work, friends. Daily we hear these words from our patients: "I can't take it anymore." "I can't live with this pain." "This isn't living—this is being alive." Many question their purpose in life when pain disrupts their major roles: "Who am I if I can no longer provide for my family?" "Who am I if I can't do the dishes, take out the garbage, tuck my kids in?" Some go further and wonder whether they still want to go on with their lives when their suffering is so great. A few have asked themselves the question: "Do I want to live or not?" Family members too are affected by the pain and suffering of their loved ones, reacting to it with resentment, sadness, guilt and hopelessness. In the face of chronic pain, many people respond with discouragement, hopelessness and helplessness.

This book is for the hundreds of people whose lives have been eroded by pain—be it the occasional migraine or backache or the ongoing intense suffering—who were told, "There is nothing more we can do for you." Our purpose is to provide you with hope and to give you tools that have worked for others. You can gain control over your pain and over your life!

This book does not give a "quick fix" or a "magic cure." Although we discuss most of the traditional and new developments in the field, the emphasis is on teaching ways to manage life with chronic pain. Pain affects not only our physical being, but our psychological functioning, including our emotions, our thinking, our behavior and our relationship to others. If pain affects all areas of life, then pain management must involve changing a way of life. Dealing with pain is inseparable from dealing with other aspects of self—emotional, mental, physical, social, sexual or spiritual. We discuss pain within the framework of a person's whole being. Also addressed are questions that are frequently asked but not dealt with when only treating the physical aspects of pain: What meaning can I find in my life? How can I cope with this crisis? Do I choose to go on living or not? And how can I make my life meaningful and worthwhile?

Our book is not intended as a substitute for a good pain management program. It however provides you with principles and guidelines on your path to health and wholeness. This book can be most effective when used in conjunction with a pain management program. It is particularly useful for psychotherapists working with persons with chronic pain and outlines a step-by-step approach—in workbook form—for the treatment of the pain patient in therapy.

The outline of the book follows the general framework of our program. We provide education and walk you through the different steps of pain management. If pain is a crisis that affects a person's whole being, not just physical aspects, then pain management needs to address all areas of a person's functioning: physical, mental, emotional, social, sexual and spiritual. The first chapter in the book discusses the psychological impact of pain. Later chapters explore different aspects of pain management. Chapter 2 describes the nature of pain because understanding how pain works helps us lower it.

Chapter 3 describes some of the frustrations encountered in typical pain management. In Chapter 4, we discuss taking charge of the pain. The next five chapters address emotional, behavioral, mental, interpersonal and spiritual aspects of pain management. At the end, we provide a review and a list of resources.

The book is intended to be used as a workbook, with space for you to write and participate. Just reading the material will not be helpful unless you actively *participate* and *apply* your learning. As we already said, this can be most effective if you use it as an adjunct to a pain management program. This book is not in lieu of a total pain program but is a good start in giving you the basic tools. If you are suffering from chronic pain, you can learn to control it and to live a full and satisfying life.

Chapter 1

The Psychological Impact of Pain

"I'm a changed man. If it weren't for my looks,
no one would know me."

Lenny*, a tall, burly, muscular man in his early forties who could be a shoe-in for Kenny Rogers, looks very much like the stereotype of the macho truckdriver which he was before the accident nearly seven years ago. Lenny's voice was animated as he described the event that changed his life: "I fell over nine feet to the ground below. I sprained my left ankle, broke the right ankle and shattered the heel. This drove my knee up, drove my hip up and injured a back injury that I had prior to that. Now my hip is messed up, my ankles are messed up, everything's messed up..."

Lenny was operated on the day after the accident where they put a steel pin in his ankle. He went to work several months following the surgery but could only last for a few months due to the pain. He went to the doctor who told him to have another operation. "They took a bone out of my hip and fused it into my ankle. They also gave me some epidural blocks for pain but I was still having trouble with the knee and I had muscle spasms which got me clear out of bed.

"I couldn't drive for long periods of time. Before the accident I was working 12 to 18 hours a day, seven days a week. But I couldn't take pain medications while I was driving so they put me where I was moving car doors. I had to do some lifting which totally messed me up. My ankle started swelling, and I couldn't take it. After only four and a half days, I called the doctor. He told me to take some more time off..." Lenny's voice trailed off.

---

*The names and some details have been changed to protect identities.

"That's the last I worked..."

Lenny described his various attempts to go back to work and the maze of doctors and treatments he went through for his pain over the past six years: "physical therapy, TENS units, cold packs, nerve blocks, pain medications, muscle spasm pills, pain pills, acupuncture, exercise.....but nothing has relieved the pain.

"My doctor told me I have traumatic muscular dystrophy or something. Although it's healed, the pain is still there. I asked him, 'Doctor, am I nuts?' He said, 'No, it's very common. Although it's healed, the brain still sends pain signals.'" Essentially, Lenny's doctors told him that there was nothing more they could do for him.

"The doctors kept suggesting medical leave but I took myself off that to go back. But I couldn't do any physical work, and I couldn't work for eight hours. In addition, I have had a learning disability and had to get tutoring for reading when I was twenty four."

Lenny became more agitated as he said: "Who the hell is going to hire someone who can't read or write, who can't sit too long, who can't stand on their feet, who can't lift, who can't do anything more than a half hour without having to lie down— would you hire someone like that?

"As far as how I spend my day now, I have a big farm with lots of animals. I get up early each morning. It takes me thirty minutes to feed the animals and water the flowers. Then I go inside and drink coffee and watch all the 'I Love Lucy' shows I can't stand. Sometimes I'll call my mother and talk to her or call my brother and we'll talk. In the afternoon, if I go outside, there's so much to do—pick up papers, sticks, truck parts, but I can't lift any heavy stuff. If I go on the tractor for twenty minutes, I need two hours to relax. I may go out for thirty minutes to an hour and a half. I don't take pain pills in the afternoon because my wife comes home, my children come home. I don't want them to see me in la la land. So I just sit and have a beer and wait for them.

"We're kind of old-fashioned—my wife's the woman of the house—I'm the man of the house. I do the cars—she does the laundry. If I feel good, I'll get up and make dinner. But if I make dinner, it will take me all day to prepare what we'll have that day. If I even go outside, then I come back too tired and have to turn off the cooking. If I cook, I can't do anything else that day. I can only go twenty to thirty minutes before I have to take a break.

"We put up a pool so I could exercise and it would help with the pain but I can't even get into the pool—my leg hurts too much. I still get up there and try—I try my level best—but when the pain gets bad, that's all I can do."

Lenny's wife, in addition to working full-time, has the bulk of the responsibilities at home. She and his children take care of the chores at night. It is all that Lenny can do to take care of himself during the day and feed the animals in the morning.

This is very different from Lenny's active life-style before the accident. "I used to have motorcycles, a dirt bike, a boat, I'd build street rods and run them up and down streets. I played basketball with my son, I 'd go fishing and hunting but only a little because I can't kill animals. We used to go bowling, we'd go to the mall and shop around. I had to sell my motorcycles because I can't ride them anymore. My wife and son won't go riding because they don't want to go without me. I can't go fishing anymore. People don't realize how many muscles you use when you use a rod. I was 165 pounds before—now I weigh 219 pounds. I can't lose it because I can't move around. I sold my boat and sold my motor home. I used to make good money but now I don't have any. The only thing I have is my wife's $130 from her job.

"Let's put it this way. This is the best way I can explain it—you'll excuse my language—I'm pissed off—*I feel I've been cheated out of life.* I've lost out on $263,000 from work in lost wages. It's hard to explain—my wife leaves for work early every morning. I watch my wife go to work and I go back and sit on my butt. I don't know anyone who'd not feel the way I do. I'm tired of saying bye bye to my wife and I go back and sit at home. The injury has let my family down.

"I'm irritable and angry all the time. I'm short-tempered with other people. I'll get angry at anybody. I'll go to the local market. If I get behind someone who's slow, I'll yell, 'Will you move the hell out of here!' I'm impatient with my wife and kids. I don't talk to anyone. You'd put six or seven people here and you'd never get a word out of me. I don't like crowds. I used to love going dancing. Now I don't even listen to country music. Why would you want to go to a dance hall and see other people dance? I won't do it. If I'm going, I'm going to dance. It's kind of like going to Pizza Hut and ordering an egg sandwich.

"My neighbor just bought a new car. My brother-in-law just bought a new car. When I was working, I bought anything I ever wanted. My brother-in-law knew how I felt. He said, 'You've done well with my sister.' But it bothers you. *I'm a changed man. If it weren't for my looks, no one would know me.*

"We used to go to the park, do regular activities. Now my friends don't even come around. Not many people want to come and sit on the couch and not do things. They want to do things. *I don't enjoy my life as I did—it's not full.*

"There's been times—I'll tell the truth here—if I felt my wife and children could go on with their life—if my wife could find someone physically able and who'd support her, I'd kill myself, I'd do it...It's crossed my mind but no, I've never put the gun to my head...it's the thought."

Pain As An Identity Crisis

Lenny's story comes in many different shades and variations. Not everyone with pain of course goes through what Lenny did, but many people are influenced to some degree or other, some only sporadically and intermittently, others on a daily basis. As you heard Lenny's story, you may have been able to identify with some of it—or your story may be very different. Whether pain affects your life very little or a lot, you may be able to relate to some aspects of Lenny's experience and benefit from some of the tools we have to help you and others with pain cope better.

For Lenny, pain is more than a physical nuisance that one has to tolerate but a factor that crosses into every aspect of his life and his feelings about himself. Lenny's pain affected the general quality of his life, his relationship with his family and friends, and his *identity*. As he himself states, "I'm a changed man." The pain crisis for Lenny was so profound that he even began to question whether his life was worth living.

Pain can be a crisis that hits at the core of one's being, at the essence of the self. Who am I if I am no longer a provider, husband, father, friend, athlete, *man*? What good am I if I can't do anything now? Pain is an identity crisis that strikes at our physical, mental, emotional and spiritual functioning. Certainly the physical losses for Lenny were very pronounced: he could no longer work or do the recreational activities he once enjoyed. He had to forego almost all the physical pursuits that both defined him as a man and that gave pleasure to his life.

His pain impinged upon his relationship with his wife and children as well. How does it feel for "an old-fashioned man" like Lenny to "wave bye bye to my wife every morning" and rely on her meager paycheck for support? How does it feel for a strong "macho" father not to be able to play basketball with his son? To take him hunting or fishing? Like many families whose loved ones experience pain, Lenny's curtailed their activities as well. If he couldn't motorcycle, boat, fish, dance or go to the mall, neither would they. So this naturally gregarious person got more and more withdrawn, avoiding friends altogether. His anger and impatience at the situation further alienated his family and friends. Lenny only hints at the marital tensions and loss in intimacy that are felt by many people with chronic pain.

The financial losses for Lenny were also great. Whereas he was able to live comfortably before, he had to curtail his lifestyle now. Lenny could calculate to the penny how much he had lost in wages. But even more significant was his feeling about himself as a provider. In a nation where one's worth is measured by one's productivity, the financial loss reflects his reduced value as a person. If I can't contribute, what good am I?

The emotional frustrations are only hinted at by Lenny. To look at the chores that need to be done and not being able to complete them, to get tired after working for only brief periods of time, to have to continuously interrupt a task to rest—what does that feel like? Lenny, like others, talks about his anger and frustration, and although he doesn't often allow himself to cry, he has bouts of depression and questions whether he should go on. He doubts the very meaning in life if he has to forego his identity.

The suffering associated with the pain only aggravates the depression. Is life worth living if I hurt so much? How can I find pleasure when I'm in so much pain? Most people can identify with feelings of pain that keep us from focusing on anything else. How can one learn to tolerate this discomfort? *Can* one do that?

Pain As Loss

For Lenny and others, pain involves loss—physical, financial and otherwise. In Lenny's case, it involved the loss of his mobility, his livelihood, his friends, his motorcycle, his boat, his motorhouse, his role as a provider, his ability to dance, fish, hunt and countless other privations. Others report losses in daily activities most people take for granted—walking, sitting, moving, lifting.

One of the biggest losses of course is the loss of health which has several components, including the ability to feel physically comfortable, to engage in "normal" activities and to see oneself as a "healthy" person. Pain first of all is a *loss of feeling good*. As many of our patients tell us, "Sometimes it gets so bad, I'll sit down and cry." Living with daily, often excruciating discomfort—and for many—the prospect of always having to tolerate this unpleasant state of affairs is more than they can stand. "It's indescribable: I can't breathe, I can't lie down, I can't focus...I cannot even begin to describe this agony and I can't imagine anything worse," said one woman. "It's like a hot searing iron all over my body." "Hell would have to be better than this." said another. "The knowledge that pain like this can come at anytime never completely leaves me, even when I'm not doubled over. I never expect to feel good..." We hear statements like this daily which only highlights this loss of feeling good.

The loss of *mobility* is another severe loss. Not being able to move your arms or legs, to walk, stand, lift or turn your head can be devastating. Many people do not even realize how many of our daily activities are affected by not being able to move even one part of the body. Sheila, a woman who hurt her neck, reports, "I can't crochet. If I even have to look up or down to see what I'm doing, it hurts. You still have to use your head. I can't hold my head long enough to wash my hair. I can't go to the grocery store because you have to look up or down. I won't drive in heavy traffic since I can't turn my head and may hit someone." Others report losses in the most routine activities that would not be considered excessively physical by most people.

Together with the loss of mobility comes the *loss of independence*. Not being able to complete a task without help, relying on others to do things for you that you used to be able to do yourself can be both humiliating and frustrating, as can be seen from these statements:

- "I can fold the laundry but I can't carry it."
- "I can vacuum on good days but I can't move the furniture. I have to wait till my husband gets home to do that for me."
- "I can start dinner but I can't stand in front of the stove while it cooks."
- "I can't wash my hair because I can't lift my arm. I have to wait for my husband to wash it for me."
- "I can go to the store but someone else has to carry the groceries for me."
- "I can't put on pantyhose without help."
- "I can't tie my shoelaces."
- "I can't clip my fingernails. I hate to rely on my wife or daughter to do that."

And on and on and on...

The *loss of a full life* is another major trauma. As Lenny stated, "I feel that I have been cheated out of life", and like him, many people with chronic pain can not engage in most of the activities they used to—be they dancing, bowling, fishing, hiking or even going to the mall. They find that they are no longer participating in the daily events that gave them pleasure and start feeling excluded from life. The loss of job and income for some can include an even more dramatic change in lifestyle. Sherry, a mother of four, reports: "This lifestyle—it stinks—it sucks—I can't get used to it. I used to work two jobs and I used to do things with the kids. I don't mean take them—I mean go *with* them. Now I can't even sit with them at the movies." Sherry continued, "This is not living—this is being alive. I don't consider it living when you can't be with your kids and do what you want to do." As Lenny said, "I don't enjoy my life as I did— *it's not full.*"

The loss of livelihood, income, standard of living, and a social life is of course more pronounced for some people than others. However, for many people with chronic pain, these reflect a *loss of role*. Lenny and Sherry both lost their roles as providers and to some extent as spouses and parents. As Sherry put it: "I get depressed when I see something in the house and I can't do it. I think, Jesus Christ, I used to work two jobs and now I can't do anything—*what good am I?*" The loss of the roles of providers, man or woman of the house, parent, can lead to the very *loss of identity*. What am I if I can't cook for my family anymore? Who am I if I can't play ball with my kids? Who am I if I can't braid my daughter's hair? Each day and with each limitation, people with chronic pain are faced with their changing identity.

Some, like Sherry and Lenny, begin to question their very value in life. Not only do they ask, "*Who* or *what* am I if I am not a provider?", they ask, "*What good* am I if I cannot pay the bills, clean the house, take my children fishing, cook dinner?" In a culture where one's worth is dependent on one's doing and contributing, this can be a very real crisis. For many, the loss of identity is also the *loss of self-worth*. Who am I now that I'm sick? How do other people see me? Many individuals with chronic pain are afraid that their identity will be that of a "sick" person and that they will be defined by their illness. This is particularly true if they are given labels like "disabled" or "invalid", together with the stigma that is associated with those epithets. They view themselves as "damaged goods", which is a further assault to their dignity as human beings.

The loss in self-esteem comes from the shame of having a body that defies control, a body that doesn't function the way you want it to. Unlike a vehicle that doesn't work, it cannot be traded for another model. To feel trapped in a body that fails you daily—is it any wonder that so many people come to feel hate and shame at this very large part of themselves? Frequently, there are also very visible changes in appearance, whether these be weight gain resulting from the inactivity as in Lenny's case, bloating from the medications, sloppy grooming from the difficulty in washing one's hair and taking care of one's hygiene, or the bodily changes that may accompany pain, be they a stiff posture, a neck brace or a limp. The insult to body image that frequently accompanies pain extends not only to one's feelings about one's attractiveness but also to seeing oneself as a sexual being. Self-love is necessary for healthy sexuality but is not easy to achieve when the body is not working properly—particularly in a society which places so much emphasis on physical fitness and bodily perfection. In a culture where self-worth is frequently defined by how "sexy" or attractive one is to the opposite sex, the cost in self-esteem can be damaging. And so, many people with chronic pain begin to question their identity. If I can't do what I am used to do, if I don't even look the way I did, who am I? What is my value?

The loss of self worth frequently is accompanied by a *loss of meaning in life*. Some ask themselves all the philosophical questions: Why me? Why is this happening? What good is living if I am suffering and in pain? What is my purpose in life if I cannot contribute? Many start questioning their basic beliefs about their purpose in life.

Not everyone with pain undergoes all these changes, of course. Some may only encounter these losses once in a while—other people may have worse experiences. However, regardless of the degree of privation, most people go through a series of stages in dealing with their loss and grief. Psychiatrist Elizabeth Kübler-Ross (1969) interviewed over 200 patients who knew they were going to die within a short time. She believed that these terminally ill patients went through a number of phases to adjust to the loss. The first stage is *denial* where people are still in shock or don't believe the bad news. This stage may serve a protective function to numb the grief. This is followed by the second stage, *anger,* when the truth can no longer be denied. The third stage is *bargaining* where the terminally ill person pleads to God or others for more time, followed by the fourth stage, *depression,* over separating from loved ones. Fifth and last is peaceful *acceptance* of the inevitable loss. Naturally, not all terminally ill people go through these stages nor necessarily in such a predictable order. Some people may not become depressed, others may not get angry and not everyone achieves acceptance. However, when dealing with any loss, be it death, divorce, loss of health, job or whatever, many people experience varying forms of these stages. Other researchers have modified some of Kübler-Ross' concepts and have included other emotions such as anxiety, guilt and panic in the grief cycle.

The "Good Grief" Cycle

Regardless of how many stages there are between the initial denial of the loss and coming to terms with it, most researchers agree that there are desirable versus undesirable ways to grieve. There is a healthy adjustment process or "Good Grief" cycle (Westberg, 1962) where learning takes place (see table on next page). This is not an easy course but any change or adjustment involves some of these phases.

Let us look at this "Good Grief" cycle*, starting with the denial of the loss and ending with a resolution of the crisis. The first reaction to a major loss is usually that of shock and denial ("This isn't really happening"). This stage does not take place overnight. There are frequently a series of steps often characterized by numerous doctor visits, medical tests and treatment where the pain is seen as a temporary disruption of our lives and there is hope that something can be done to get rid of it for once and for all. Of course for many people—those with temporary acute pain—that is often the case. When the pain lingers, when one has to face that the underlying problem may never go away, that the illness has become one's normal condition—then one begins the grieving process. The initial denial and detachment when reality hasn't sank in has a protective function and can numb us to the painful feelings that then follow.

---

*Adapted from Donald A. Tubesing's Stress Skills workshop presented in Phoenix, Arizona, 1978.

The Good Grief Cycle

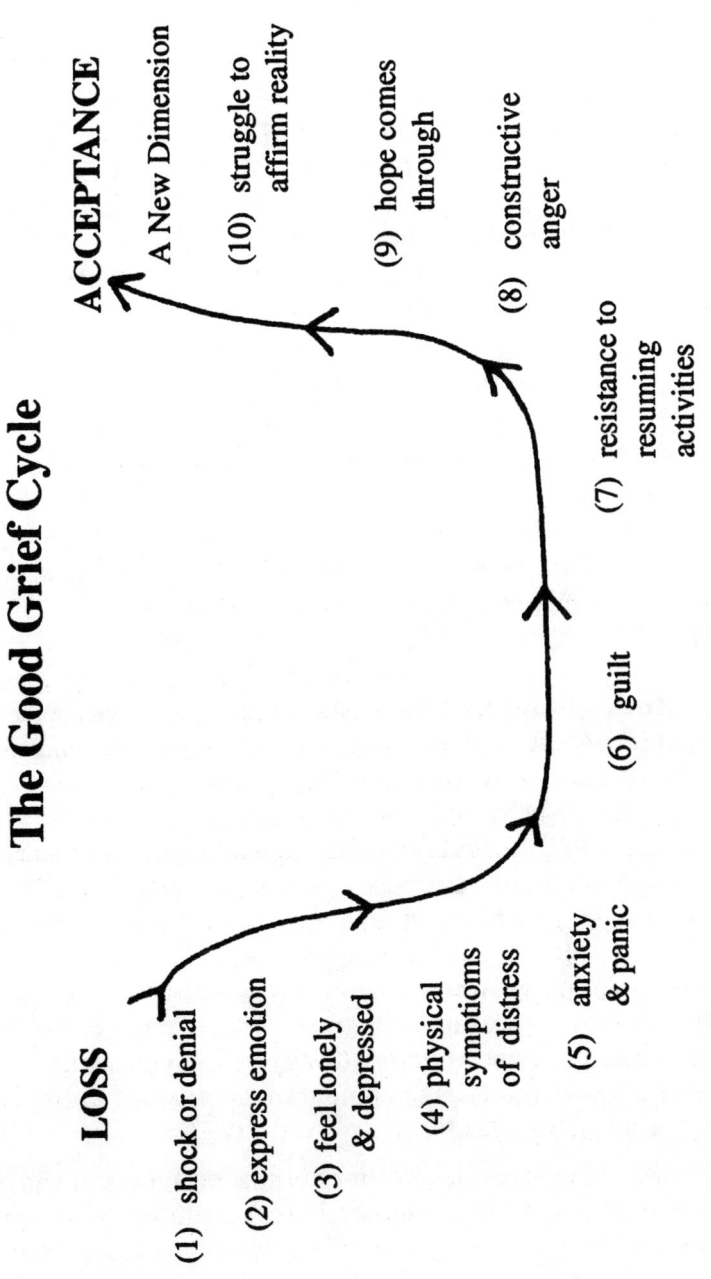

LOSS

(1) shock or denial

(2) express emotion

(3) feel lonely & depressed

(4) physical symptioms of distress

(5) anxiety & panic

(6) guilt

(7) resistance to resuming activities

(8) constructive anger

(9) hope comes through

(10) struggle to affirm reality

ACCEPTANCE

A New Dimension

The denial not only takes the form of detachment from distressing feelings but also refusing to accept physical limitations, often at the cost of further wear and tear on the body. ("I have always been athletic and I am not going to let this change my routine" or "It is not really hurting"). The denial stage is not a one time event: it happens over and over again, and persons with chronic pain frequently discount their bodily restrictions. We will be talking later on about how this denial can lead to them constantly pushing their bodies further than they can go and having to deal with the unpleasant consequences afterwards.

Once some of the initial shock of the injury wears off and the realization hits that this isn't going to go away, once the get well cards, flowers and visitors stop, there can be a variety of emotions in accommodating to the reality. Sadness and depression are a natural reaction to loss and some mourning is necessary before "biting the bullet" and moving on. Sometimes other physical symptoms appear in reaction to the loss which can unfortunately increase the level of subjective pain. People who "stuff their feelings" may manifest other physical symptoms of distress as ulcers, headaches and general bodily tensions. Anxiety and panic are also common to loss with one feeling that somehow he or she is to blame for the pain. We frequently hear statements like, "My body has let me down" or as Lenny said, "My injury has let my family down." Individuals with pain also feel guilt at not being able to do things they could, at being dependent on others, and some may even feel that they must have done something wrong to deserve this suffering. There is a resistance to resuming new activities or going back to old activities if one cannot engage in them fully. For example, Lenny stopped listening to country music which he loved because he can't dance anymore ("Why would you want to go to a dance hall and see other people dance? I *won't* do it! If I'm going, I'm going to dance").

Constructive anger is another necessary aspect of the good grief cycle. Many persons get stuck in this phase because they are unable to express their anger directly at the source. Instead, they displace it to the people who are "safe"— usually their families. Being impatient and short-tempered is very characteristic of many people with pain. Unfortunately, this only further alienates and isolates them from their loved ones. Some people in pain lash out at the "system"—blaming their doctors for their predicament and because they cannot help them. We will describe the patient-doctor interaction later on in the book. Persons involved in litigation have even more anger to hold on to which frequently only aggravates the pain and may get them stuck in the "bad grief" cycle. We will discuss constructive versus destructive ways of expressing anger in later chapters. However, healthy anger—anger that heals—is a natural part of resolving the crisis and reaching acceptance.

There is no precise timetable for grieving over the loss of one's health. When you have lost a part of you, it is no different than grieving for a friend or a loved one. You need to mourn on your own schedule and in your own way. Many people do not want to be seen as engaging in self-pity, and indeed there may be a fine line between a self-absorbing preoccupation with the loss and healthy grieving but too many individuals prematurely forego the stages between denial and acceptance, often encouraged by others to "just face it and go on with your life".

By dealing with the different phases and emotions of the pain crisis, one is able to experience hope again and learn to let go, achieving a new level of acceptance. Many people are able to find ways to accommodate physical pain without either denying its reality or letting it take over their lives. If grief can run its natural course, it eventually abates although it is never over for once and for all, just as we don't stop grieving for a loved one. However, we can learn not to be so engulfed in grief that it robs us of enjoying life again.

Crisis has been defined (by Webster) as a "turning point in the course of a situation" and a "situation whose outcome decides whether possible bad consequences will follow". The Chinese symbol for crisis has two components: danger and opportunity. Every crisis or loss has within it the potential for learning from it and for rising above it. We will discuss this more fully in a later section. One of the aims of this book is to help you with this process.

Taking Stock: Where Are You Now?

To guide you through the stages of grief, take a few minutes to reflect on the particular losses you have experienced as a result of the pain. Some losses could be intense and pervade all aspects of your life; others could be less dramatic.

Write down these losses in the spaces below:

Losses I Have Experienced As a Result of Pain:

_____

_____

_____

_____

_____

_____

_____

_____

_____

_____

_____

_____

_____

_____

_____

_____

_____

_____

Now take a look at the table (The "Good Grief" Cycle) on page 11 again.

Study those stages and circle those which have been particularly difficult for you, those in which you have gotten "stuck".

(1) Which stages have been particularly difficult for me?

_____

_____

_____

_____

_____

_____

_____

(2) What are some of the ways that I keep myself stuck? Describe those ways. (For example, "I still vacuum even though it always lays me up for a few days afterwards. That is denying I have limitations" or "I yell at my kids when I am really angry at the situation".)

_____

_____

_____

_____

_____

_____

_____

_____

_____

_____

_____

_____

_____

3)   What are some ways I have used to get out of such stages?

_____

_____

_____

_____

_____

_____

_____

_____

_____

_____

_____

(4)   What are some strengths that I have to offer myself and others because of my pain crisis?

_____

_____

_____

_____

_____

_____

   The last two questions are only to get you started to think about coping tools that you already have. These are open-ended lists and you will add to them as you proceed with your program.

Where Do You Want To Be?

You have had a chance to look at how your pain has affected your life and which of the stages of the "good grief" cycle you are at. Now we would like you to think about where you would like to go from here. To help you with this process, we will ask you the "Miracle Question". If you went to sleep and woke up the next morning and a miracle were to happen during the night, so that your pain stopped but you still had the same physical limitations, how would your life be different when you woke up? Aside from not hurting, what else would change? What would you do differently? How would you feel about yourself? What would your relationship be like with others? How would your thoughts and behaviors be? Write down exactly what would happen—not just, for example, "My pain will go away" or "My outlook would be better" but "I would smile at my husband", "I would invite some friends for dinner", "I would look in the mirror and like what I saw", "I would laugh at jokes", "I would listen to music", etc. Focus on what you would do and how you would behave. When you describe how your "miracle" will be, do so realistically within the limits of your situation. Just as one cannot expect a middle-aged person for example to look like or have the same stamina as an adolescent, we cannot set expectations that are not realistic for us. You cannot change reality—an injured back remains an injured back—but *you can reduce your pain dramatically so that you feel good.* You may still have to circumscribe your activities to some extent—but you can do those activities enjoyably and comfortably in a relatively pain-free manner.

You may wish to use the following list to further help you clarify your goals. Let us look at some realistic goals. Check those that fit for you and add others that are not included here.

☐   1. to reduce pain and feel physically more comfortable

☐   2. to return to my usual role in daily life

☐   3. to return to work

☐   4. to increase my independence

☐   5. to feel useful

☐   6. to learn ways to cope with pain

- [ ] 7. to decrease my medications
- [ ] 8. to increase my physical activity and endurance
- [ ] 9. to reduce my pain behaviors, e.g. those that draw attention to my pain and result in increased pain for me
- [ ] 10. to improve my relationship with my family
- [ ] 11. to sleep better
- [ ] 12. to be less depressed
- [ ] 13. to enjoy life more
- [ ] 14. to feel more in control of my life
- [ ] 15. to enhance my sexual functioning
- [ ] 16. to feel better about myself and my body
- [ ] 17. to be less irritable
- [ ] 18. to have a more rewarding social life

19. _____

20. _____

21. _____

22. _____

23. _____

24. _____

25. _____

Pain Management As A Way of Life: What Can I Do About My Pain?

We have seen how chronic pain can impinge on almost every aspect of ourselves as persons. Since pain affects all of you, not just your arm, leg or back, then managing your pain must deal with all parts of your life, not just the physical, as can be seen from the chart on the next page.

Managing your pain is managing your life. Since pain has a direct bearing on your emotional, social and spiritual well-being, then a pain program for you would have to address all those factors. Pain management is looking at *the person as a whole.*

PAIN MANAGEMENT AS A WAY OF LIFE

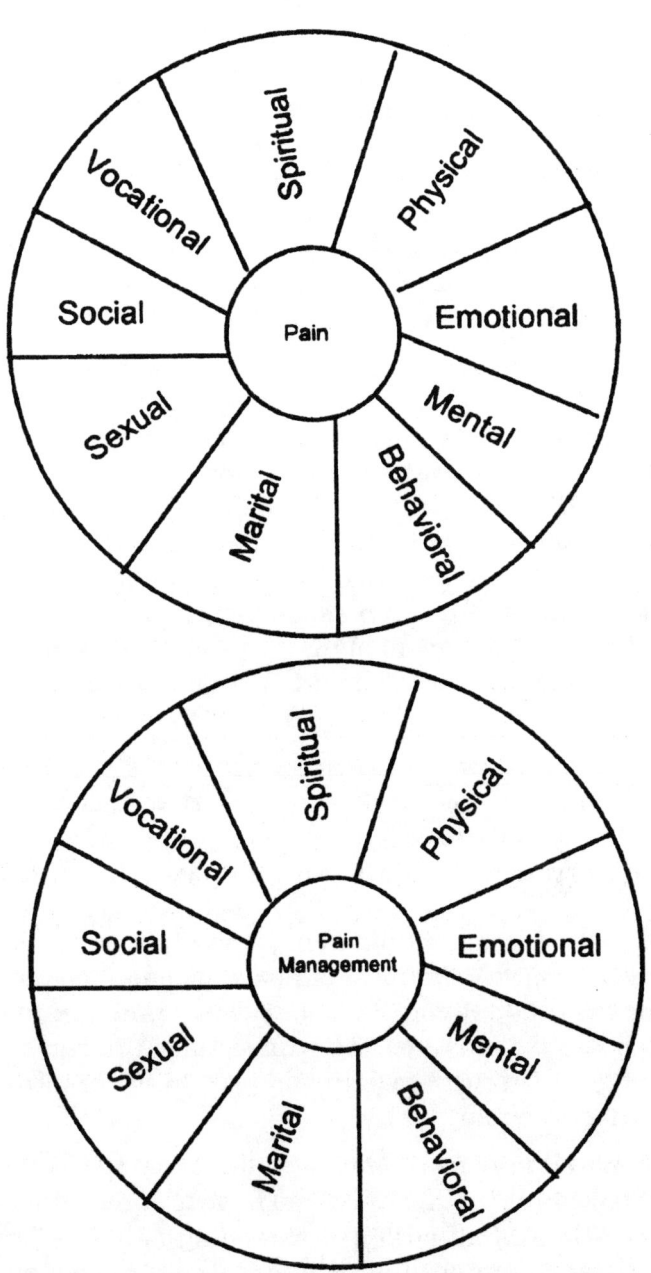

Pain management is a daily undertaking. It is not a one-time "quick fix". Many people with chronic pain are still looking for the magic pills or the treatment that will magically "cure" their condition for once and for all. Unfortunately, that does not often happen. Pain management is *comprehensive* and is a combination of many different treatment modalities. We will outline these in a later chapter. Pain management is also a *daily* commitment, not a one-time event that takes care of the problem for once and for all. Just as maintaining healthy teeth and a well-toned body requires daily flossing and exercise, so does keeping yourself pain-free require daily work. A healthy set of teeth or a conditioned body does not happen overnight but necessitates *continuous monitoring.*

Pain management is also pain prevention. Preventing your pain from getting out of control requires ongoing care. You cannot trade in your body for a new model if it doesn't function the way it used to, as you can a car. If you are going to have this model for life, then it will require non-stop attention to let it remain in the best shape it can be. It means frequently checking it, not taking it on long trips if it can't handle them and not running it to the ground. It means constant upkeep to stave off a breakdown. Similarly, in managing your pain, you will need to take preventive steps to avert further breakdown of your parts.

Pain management requires your active participation in your treatment. Your doctors and other health providers can help but they can't do it all. You have to do at least 90% of the work and you have to do it on a daily basis. Taking personal responsibility for taking care of yourself provides you with a sense of control, that you can help yourself. It keeps you from feeling like a *victim,* a helpless puppet dependent on the whims of fate or the gods. It may be true that you cannot undo tissue damage but you *can* reduce the pain signal. You can also take charge of how you react to pain and learn ways to minimize it and its effects on your life.

Although it may feel to you as it did to Lenny that the pain has cheated you out of life, you do not have to *allow* it to continue to do so. When faced with overwhelming pain, we have two choices: to let it dominate our lives or to learn to deal with it so that we are in control. Most people in their more rational moments would choose the latter. Living with pain does not mean "giving up" or "giving in". It doesn't mean, as one woman said, "I might just as well sit down and die." Dealing with pain is not a passive stance but an *active* taking charge. If pain is going to be a part of my life, I have to know this companion and co-exist with it. Taking charge of your pain means, first of all, learning about pain in general and yours in particular, acquiring tools to cope with it and to prevent it from getting out of hand, and being a very active participant in your care and treatment.

Dr. Bernie Siegel (1986) in his book *Love, Medicine and Miracles* reports that he sees three kinds of patients. About 15 to 20% have given up on life and may even welcome illness as an escape. About 60 or 70%, the majority of patients, are in the middle, those who act the way the doctors want them to act and who hope that the doctor will do all the work, who "given a choice, would rather be operated on than actively work to get well." The remainder, roughly 15 to 20%, are what Siegel terms "exceptional patients". Those refuse to play the victim. Although these are frequently difficult and challenging patients because they demand their rights, ask questions, get second opinions and do not easily submit, they are also the most likely group to get well.

What kind of patient are you?

_____

_____

_____

_____

_____

_____

Do you believe that you have control over the rewards in your life or do you believe that chance, luck or fate pay a large role in what happens to you? Take a few minutes to respond to the following questions:

Use a choice for each item. In some cases you will find that you believe both statements or neither one. Please make a decision anyway.

1. a. I often find myself saying something or doing something to the effect of "What will be will be."
   b. I believe that what happens to me is my own doing.
2. a. I deserve credit for most of my accomplishments.
   b. I've been fortunate to have done well on a number of occasions.
3. a. I'm a pretty confident person. I can make things happen.
   b. Sometimes I'm amazed at how things seem to happen to me all by themselves.
4. a. I feel like a Ping-Pong ball. Life just bounces me back and forth between happy and sad.
   b. If I want to be happy, I just choose a fun thing to do and go to it.
5. a. I plan things, and they turn out as I expect.
   b. "Come what may," that's my motto. I'm a tumbleweed caught in the wind.
6. a. In this country, anyone with some talent and some sweat is going to make it.
   b. If you're lucky, you're rich: if not, join the crowd.
7. a. Sometimes I feel powerful, able to do whatever I want.
   b. Sometimes I feel powerless, the victim of mysterious forces.

Give yourself a point if you choose each of the following alternatives: 1.a; 2.b.; 3.b.; 4.a; 5.b.; 6.b.;7.b. The higher the score, the more external you are. What is your score?_____

Based on C.R. Potkey and B.P. Allen (1986)

This is a scale on *locus of control* (Rotter, 1972) which measures differences in beliefs about how much we can control the good or bad things that happen to us in life. The scale divides people into *internals* who believe they have control over the rewards in their lives and *externals* who believe chance and powerful other people control their lives.

Most people do not of course fall neatly into one category or the other. Research has shown that in situations where people do have control over what happens to them, e.g.,school, work, etc., it usually pays for them to have an internal locus of control. However, in situations where they really do not have control, internals become extremely frustrated whereas externals just go with the flow. What does this mean for you? It means being realistic about what you can change and what you can't: changing what you can control and learning to accept what you can't control. You may not be able to change the structural damage to your body—a broken back is a broken back—but you can reduce the pain signal so that you are not as uncomfortable. You can lower your pain dramatically so that you can feel good. You also have a great deal of control in how much you allow it to rule your life.

Accepting personal responsibility and taking an active role in your management is not the same as taking the blame for your pain as many people are prone to do. You may think that if I can help myself get well, then I must have been responsible for getting ill in the first place. Unnecessary guilt serves no function and only intensifies what you are already going through. You did not *cause* your pain but you can learn to control it.

Learning to live with pain involves conscious choice. The choice is not *if* but *how* we accept pain. "No matter how philosophical you are, pain is never really acceptable" someone told us. "I don't have to *accept* it but I have to learn to *take* it." The choice of how we accept pain is how much we allow it to dominate our lives.

The main message in this chapter is that of hope when you recognize that you can play a very large part in managing your pain. You do not feel so powerless when you learn that you can do a great deal about it. To make informed decisions, to feel in control, you first of all need education—education about pain in general, your own pain and tools to manage your pain and your life.

In the next few chapters, we will guide you through this educational process. We will discuss the aspects of pain so that it will not seem so mysterious, we will provide you with information about treatments for pain management and we will supply you with tools to control and lower your pain and the areas in your life that are affected by it. As you go through the different exercises in the book, you will apply these principles to yourself and learn to lower your pain and achieve control over your well-being. Good Luck!

Chapter 2

The Nature of Pain

"I divide the experience of pain into three stages. First there is the pain signal, an alarm that goes off when nerve endings in the periphery sense danger.......At the second stage of pain, the spinal cord and base of the brain act as a "spinal gate" to sort out which of the many millions of signals deserve to be forwarded as a message to the brain.......The final stage of pain takes place in the higher brain...which sorts through the prescreened messages and decides on a response. Indeed, pain does not truly exist until the entire cycle of signal, message, response has been complete."

Paul Brand, M.D. & Philip Yancey
Pain: *The Gift Nobody Wants*

We would like to make three major points about pain. First, pain is real and in the nervous system. Secondly, pain is a signal of warning and danger. Third, pain is not the same as tissue damage.

Pain is Real and in the Nervous System

Pain is very real. You know that, and we don't need to convince you of it. Many of you may have heard that your pain is imaginary, that you're exaggerating it or that "it can't be that bad." If your injury has healed, if the tissue damage cannot be seen, then it must be "all in your head." Just because we cannot view pain doesn't mean it doesn't exist. Pain may last for years after damaged tissues have healed.

Pain is a Signal of Warning & Danger

Pain tells us that something is wrong. If we didn't feel pain, we would not know to take our hands off a hot stove before we burn ourselves further, we would not realize that we have broken a bone or cut our finger, we would not recognize if we were having a heart attack or an ear infection. Pain warns us that there is something wrong and enables us to do something about it before further damage occurs.

Ironically, not being able to feel pain can cause some serious damage. Without pain sensation, people can—and have—injured themselves because they didn't have a signal to warn them of danger. Pain is a necessity that signals a physical condition needing attention.

Pain Is Not The Same As Tissue Damage

Pain is a very strange phenomenon. Whereas it would only seem logical that pain should be directly related to physical damage, this does not appear to be the case. The most dramatic example of this occurred during the Civil War when hundreds of soldiers whose legs were amputated still felt pain in their legs *when they had no legs.* This phantom limb pain is very real even though it has no physical cause. It would appear that pain is more complex than originally thought and that it may be in our memory bank even when its original cause is removed.

Another strange phenomenon occurred during World War II which related to this aspect of pain: soldiers with severe war injuries asked for very little pain medication whereas civilians in the U.S. with similar injuries resulting from automobile accidents needed a great deal of pain medication. Doctors were puzzled as to how to explain that. How could the same tissue damage be experienced as very painful by the civilians and not by the soldiers? People in different settings experience pain differently. For the soldiers, the injury provided a relief ("I'm going to live"). They were going to go home instead of die at war. For the civilians, the injuries disrupted their lives and caused more stress. It appears then that it is not only the extent of the injury that determines the extent of the pain.

If pain serves as a signal of bodily damage, it would be expected that once the injury heals, the pain would go away. This fortunately often occurs with acute pain: once the body heals, the pain disappears. Chronic pain, however, is not necessarily associated with tissue damage. Pain and healing are not always in concert.

What Is Chronic Pain?

We need to distinguish between chronic and acute pain. Acute pain is usually sudden and occurs with an acute injury such as a broken arm. It is short-term and goes away readily once the condition is treated. Chronic pain, on the other hand, lasts much longer. It has been defined as pain that lasts greater than four to six weeks by some and greater than six months by others. Whether six weeks or six months, chronic pain is pain that lasts longer than it should. It is pain that is not necessarily connected with identifiable tissue damage, for which there is no clear-cut treatment and that lasts much longer than the expected healing period for the condition. Chronic pain, as we have seen, also involves a significant change in lifestyle, including decreased activity, loss of employment, loss of self-esteem, depression and a general feeling of lack of control over one's life. It is frequently associated with emotional and behavioral changes. This book is primarily intended for the person with chronic pain. Take a few minutes to answer yes or no to the following questions to assess whether you have chronic pain.

Do You Have Chronic Pain?

- Has your pain lasted more than six months?_____
- Has your pain lasted longer than what is normally expected for your condition? _____
- Have you tried many different types of treatment with no relief?_____
- Has your life been affected drastically by the pain?_____
- Have your feelings about yourself changed?_____
- Are you depressed?_____
- Do you find yourself getting irritable frequently?_____
- Has your relationship with your family been affected by the pain?_____
- Has your relationship with your friends been affected?_____
- Has your activity level changed dramatically?_____
- Have you been more dependent on medications to keep you going?_____
- Has your sleep been affected by the pain?_____
- Do you feel out of control frequently?_____

How Does Pain Work?

The first theory of pain, the bell theory, states simply that when there is tissue damage, it sends a direct signal to the brain, much like the ringing of a doorbell, so that the pain is felt. This is also referred to as the telephone pole theory so that when there is an injury, the nerves carry the message to the brain where it is perceived as pain when the bell rings. We can sometimes cut the telephone wire so that the message doesn't get through and the bell doesn't ring. Similarly, a dentist can numb the jaw when doing surgery so that the signal from the jaw does not reach the brain and therefore, no pain is experienced.This theory explains some aspects of pain but does not account for phantom limb pain or why similar tissue damage can bring different feelings of pain in different people. In 1965, two scientists by the name of Melzach and Wall introduced the gate control theory of pain. They said that there is a gate in the spinal cord, and when this gate is open, all the signals come through and we experience the pain. When the gate is closed, as when the dentist uses novocaine, we feel no pain. The less open the gate, the less pain we feel.

The gate control theory sees pain as having three stages. The simple statement, "my hand hurts" involves a series of steps. First, among the many scratches, sensations and irritations on my hand, very few achieve the intensity required to send a *pain signal.* This signal may or may not pass the spinal gate and be forwarded to the brain as a brain *message.* And even if it does get through the gate, it may be suppressed by the higher brain. If the pain message is not thwarted by the higher brain, then it can provoke a *response* in the brain—I will feel the pain in my hand.

The following diagram depicts this three stage process of *signal—message—response.* As can be seen from the diagram, although there is some tissue damage where the damage site is, the pain *signals* may never go through the pain gate. Even if they go through the gate, they can also be filtered from never reaching the brain *(message).* The brain can also filter these signals so that the pain is not felt *(response),* as indicated by the downward arrows from the brain.

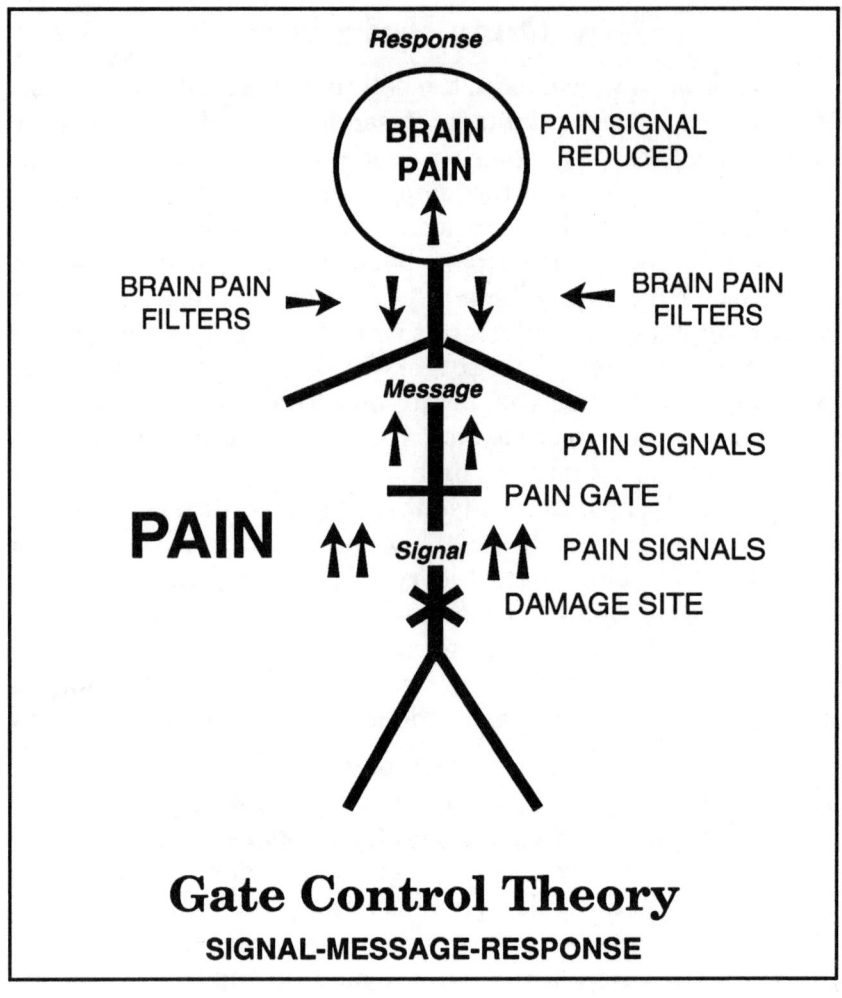

Gate Control Theory
SIGNAL-MESSAGE-RESPONSE

What regulates the gate? Some people think that endorphins, chemicals that are released from brain cells, act like morphine and inhibit pain through pathways between the brain and spinal cord. Scientists have found that the camel—the animal that is least sensitive to pain—has more endorphins than others. So the brain may have its own pain reducing chemical, and endorphins may be the action in the opening and closing of the gate.

Knowing how pain works can help you in managing your pain. Pain can be increased and decreased in intensity by opening or closing the nerve pathways from the site of the injury to the brain. Pain treatment consists of identifying the cause of the pain to know what the problem is as best as possible. The pain signal can be reduced by one or more of the following procedures as is appropriate for your medical problem. Surgery, physical therapy and anti-inflammatory medication can all intervene in the pain cycle by freeing nerves, relaxing muscles or creating more room around the nerves. You can also jam and reduce pain signals through nerves by ice packs, nerve blocks, pain medication, and TENS (Transcutaneous Electrical Nerve Stimulation) units to block and disrupt pain signals. Relaxation, medical hypnosis and biofeedback can also help the brain filter out and block pain signals. Pacing of activities can prevent the pain from getting out of control, and stress reduction can help further reduce the pain signals. In short, treatment can intervene in all stages of the pain response cycle. Understanding the ways in which pain can be filtered can help you learn ways of keeping the pain gate closed. We will talk about the various forms of treatment in more detail in later chapters. Understanding pain is a first step in learning how to manage it and seeing why your active participation is crucial for success.

Summary

Here are some of the major points we would like you to remember about pain:

1. Pain is real and in the nervous system.
2. Pain is a signal of warning and danger.
3. Pain travels from the injured site to the brain.
4. We become aware of pain when the signal reaches the brain.
5. Pain is not the same as tissue damage.
6. Pain can be increased and decreased in intensity by opening and closing the nerve pathways from the site of the injury to the brain.
7. Pain treatment consists of ways of reducing or jamming the pain signal.
8. Your active participation in this process is the key to success.

Chapter 3

Getting Help

"Doctors are busy playing God when so few
of us have the qualifications. And besides,
the job is taken."
Bernie S. Siegel, M.D.

We would have liked to start this section by telling you about the ideal treatment program for pain—one that addresses the whole person and uses an integrated multidisciplinary approach to deal with the many different aspects of pain—physical, emotional, social and otherwise. Unfortunately, what frequently happens is that people go through many different doctors and different treatments before they come to a pain center. By the time we see many of our patients, they have already consulted dozens and dozens of doctors and specialists, they are at the end of their insurance dollars rather than at the beginning—and they frequently feel like they are at the end of their rope as well. They are angry, bitter and frustrated.

Looking for the "Magic Pill"

What frequently happens is that the patient is still geared to the acute nature of the problem and is looking for a "quick fix", the magic pill or remedy that will make the pain go away. So is the physician who also does not want to deal with a problem that is chronic and not responding to traditional treatment. The patient is placed in a predicament and becomes more and more frustrated. Patients keep looking for the right doctor who will finally find the magic formula and they keep getting rejected, particularly if they have already had a history of going to dozens of specialists, and get labelled as hypochondriacs. Sometimes patients feel so defeated, they give up on the medical profession altogether and go to alternative methods of health and healing. Although they may be helped by these methods, they have cut themselves off from the potential benefits of traditional medicine.

Physicians too become very flustered when their patients don't get better. They may feel that they are not being good doctors, and of course, their patients' anger at them only reinforces this perception. They become more and more threatened and get angry at those patients who complain all the time and don't get better. They are frustrated because there are no "objective" findings. They find it hard to admit that maybe they don't know everything there is to know about the patient's situation. "If these remedies I have work for other patients and not for this one, then, of course, there must be something wrong with this patient for his or her inability feel better", they reason. "If we don't see it, it must not be there", they think, and so they tell the patient, "It's all in your head."

Patients too start to wonder if they are imagining things. If the doctors can't diagnose it, then they begin to lose hope. They either start to lose their confidence in the medical profession or they begin to doubt themselves ("It must be my imagination"). As we saw in the first chapter, even Lenny asked his doctor: "Doctor, am I nuts?" Sometimes living with self-doubt can be easier than mistrusting their physicians because if their doctors can't do anything for them, what hope is there? So it is easier to believe that the symptoms aren't "real" or that they are a "figment of my imagination" than "nobody can help me." Doctors may encourage those doubts: it is often a lot more comfortable to believe their patient is making up symptoms than to admit that maybe they are stumped. So the labels continue and get passed on from doctor to doctor, and the charts get thicker and thicker.

Patients and doctors begin to see each other as adversaries rather than partners, with each trying to prove the other wrong. Many doctors already have a predetermined conception of what their patients are like before they even examine them and may convey a hostile attitude. Patients as well may come with a chip on their shoulders when they see the next physician. Being so concerned that doctors will see them as "crazy", they will not even discuss material that may have any emotional overlay because that will confirm that "it's all in my head." As we shall see in later chapters, although stress, emotions and other factors play a very big role in opening and shutting the pain gate and in making the pain worse, admitting to stress, depression, fears or marital problems does not mean you are crazy. Unfortunately those issues are very important in the treatment of pain, and by denying or minimizing them, patients may cut themselves off from treatment that may be very helpful.

In addition, patients may magnify their pain and call attention to it in a very dramatic fashion to further prove to their health care providers how terrible the pain truly is. They will engage in frequent pain behaviors, such as grimacing, wincing, moaning and complaining, believing that the louder they complain, the more seriously they will be taken. Some patients may put on performances that would put Meryl Streep to shame, thinking that if they could only *show* how bad it really was, then they would be taken seriously. Unfortunately, just the opposite occurs. If doctors feel that you are being overly dramatic, then they think you must be acting, and that the pain must not be real. They will discount you and figure you must not be telling the truth. For example, patients are frequently asked to rate their pain on a scale of 0 to 10, with 10 being the limit. Many patients, wanting to emphasize the seriousness of their pain, will rate their pain as "eleven" when ten is the maximum on the scale. When asked where it hurts, they say "everywhere". When asked when, they reply "all the time". When queried about when it gets better, they state "never". Unfortunately, this strategy often backfires, and their credibility becomes questionable . Doctors then reason that if this person is exaggerating, then he or she must not have any pain at all. The physician will feel that the patient is crying wolf and will ignore and discount any further cries of pain.

Not only that but the doctor is unable to help because he or she is not getting accurate information. Doctors and other health care providers are paid consultants. They are there to help you with the information that is given them. Would one go to an accountant or financial manager to manage one's finances without telling that person all the facts about one's financial situation? How can that professional make a plan without having accurate information? Most people would not dream of going to an accountant and providing only vague answers as "a lot", "all the time" or "never". Not only would the accountant refuse to work with them, the IRS would not accept their statements! However, they think nothing of going to a health care provider and providing vague statements—which may get them sympathy at most but no practical help.

Rather than see the doctor as a helper or consultant, patients start seeing him or her as an adversary and try to prove to this enemy that they are not crazy, often at the cost of their own well-being. The battle lines are drawn, and other people get into the battle as well—families, insurance companies, attorneys—one side to prove that the patient is crazy, the other to prove that the doctor is incompetent. Rather than working together, they work against each other—and both sides lose. Rather than working in tandem in a position where both sides win, there are only losers in this game.

Pain Games

Norman Shealy (1976) describes the games doctors and patients play in his book *The Pain Game,* a game which can be expensive and emotionally wrenching and a game in which there are no winners. Some of the games that patients play are not necessarily in their self-interest. One of the games involved in trying to prove their sanity and to get back at the adversary is "Try to cure me if you can." Although the aim of this game is to prove the doctor is a "quack", the obvious self-defeating nature of the game results in maintaining the symptoms. You have to remain in pain in order to win at this game.

As Shealy states, "Regardless of the origin of his pain, the patient may discover that there are coincidental, secondary rewards for suffering or that his pain provides a handle with which he can manipulate others. Those games may be strong enough to keep him from recovering and he may find it worth his while to keep the pain game going" (p.4). Some of the rewards may be getting some admiration for the suffering ("I don't know how you do it"), getting out of unpleasant situations, or getting attention from others. As George Bernard Shaw has said: "I enjoy convalescence. It is the part that makes the illness worthwhile." One unfortunate secondary reward is how commonly many patients may become addicted or habituated to drugs and may use the pain to obtain narcotics from their physicians. Litigation can also serve inadvertently as a reward for pain where the financial settlement depends on the extent of the pain.

It is not only patients but doctors too that participate in this pain game. The most obvious game of course is the "It's all in your head" game. Another name for this game might be "How dare you challenge my authority!" The reasoning behind this is "I know best. If you don't benefit from what I have to offer and you get angry at me, then *you* must be *crazy.* If you are not responding to my treatment, then there must be something wrong with you."

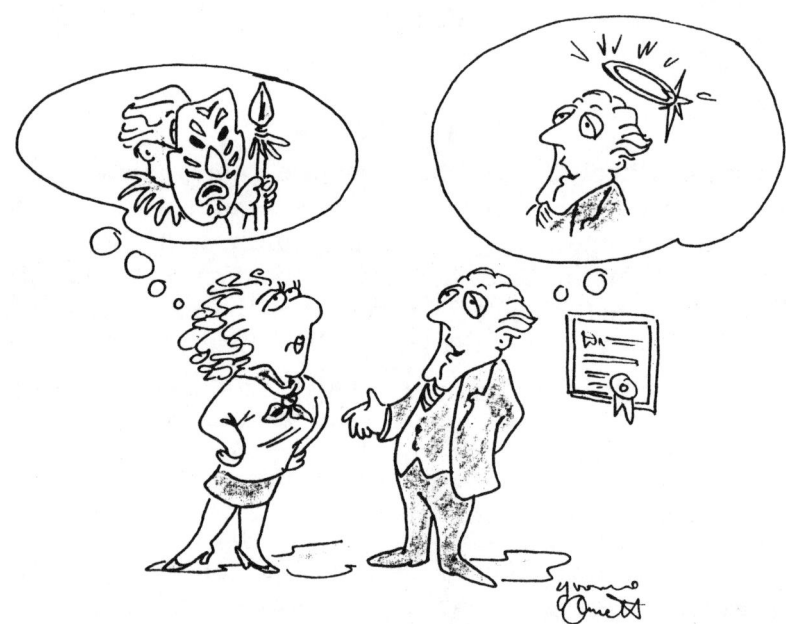

Some doctors *label* their patients and imply there is something terribly wrong with them, calling them immature, histrionic and difficult, implying it's "all in their head". The following are some excerpts from an evaluation made on patients who had documented injuries:

■ "Outside of the *alleged* 'pain' that the patient is discussing in vague terms, which may have origins prior to the injury, I see no evidence....."

■ "Mr. ___ may be self-centered and immature or childish. He may seek attention and avoid responsibility, in part through somatic symptoms. The most significant concerns related to histrionic personality features are as follows. There are signs of lassitude and malaise. He often feels uncomfortable and not in good health....I believe that it is secondary gain that is serving to maintain Mr. ___'s manifold physical, neurologic, and psychiatric symptoms. *The most effective means of treating these symptoms would therefore be to remove the source of secondary gain.*"

■ "The test results suggest that Ms. ___'s problems are primarily emotional given the absence of objective medical findings.....although the patient is compliant, she continues to have complaints on a frequent basis....*this patient will not benefit from any further medical intervention.*"

■ "I do not feel that I can provide this patient with any additional care. It is my feeling that her anger which is quite persistent....*precludes her from making any additional progress.*"

■ "Given the small amount of trauma initially inciting these symptoms, I think it is reasonable to assume that *her symptom should have been resolved at this time.* I am impressed today with the significant *psychological overlay*, i.e., anger and some elements of depression which seem to characterize her presentation."

■ "I also explained...that it is the opinion that she may return to work. She was quite upset. She told me that she wondered how anybody could expect her to work when a lot of people's lives are dependent on the quality of her work that she does and that she can't maintain the quality if she is in pain. She states she will go to a lawyer."

The battle has only just begun!

These statements only hint at how many practitioners fight the pain game. They are angry at the patients because they complain, because they are angry and they fight anger with anger. We'll get even! We'll cut off their benefits! We'll declare them well and send them back to work! That will show them! Or they write them off: "Her anger precludes her from making further progress." At any rate, whether the anger on the doctor's part is conscious or unconscious, it comes through in the clinical reports. Basically, what they are saying is that these people are unpleasant to be around, they are angry and complaining and they don't respond by the book, and we don't want to deal with them.

Part of the doctor game is a de-humanitization of the patients. Although they may not label their patients "crazy" or "histrionic", they will talk about "syndromes" rather than about people, whether they are referring to "the back in Room 18" or "renal failure in Room 22". They will also refer to them as though they were adversaries rather than co-partners: "Watch out for those patients", they tell others, "they'll take up all your time if you let them." Seeing the patient as a product, a collection of parts rather than a human being, of course only intensifies the destructive cycle of the pain game.

A variation of the "it's all in your head" game is the "you're too stupid to understand" game. Thus many physicians will not explain all the complications or risks of certain procedures. Ilene, a professional woman with a Master's degree, related specifically how this game was played. "The physician either talked *above* me using medical terms I had never heard of or *below* me, as though I were some sort of idiot who couldn't be trusted. I had written down all the medications I was taking but he ignored me and asked me to bring the bottles so he could read them himself.

"He also talked *about* me as though I weren't even there. When another doctor came in, a resident, they started conversing about me in my presence as though I were a specimen. He would ask me a question, and as I was trying to answer, he would cut me off and talk to the other doctor about my condition."

The games played by physicians are not limited to doctors of course but to other health professionals as well. Most of us, whether we are patients or health professionals or both, may feel a little uncomfortable reading some of these sections as we recognize parts of these behaviors in ourselves. Most of us can relate to and see aspects of these behaviors in us. Fortunately, most patients and health care professionals do not engage in those games. It is true that there are patients who lie about their symptoms but the research shows that only a minuscule number of people are either consciously lying or having imaginary pains. Most patients are trying very hard to find relief, and if there are emotional aspects that exacerbate the pain, that is part of the picture. There are also unfortunately a few providers who are sometimes referred to as "whores" by the legal profession who frequently work for insurance companies and who will say anything about the patients they examine to defend their case. Fortunately, these are rare too, but they can cause significant damage. All we can say about them is that they have to live with themselves and recognize the consequences of their behaviors. Most patients and providers are conscientious people trying to do a good job who are frustrated by pain that doesn't respond to traditional treatment.

Whether we are patients, providers or both, it is important that we recognize these attitudes and behaviors within ourselves that promote an adversarial position rather than a collaborative effort.

If you are a health care provider, ask yourself the following questions:

1. Have I ever taken out my frustration on a patient because he or she is not getting better?
2. Have I labelled a patient a hypochondriac because he or she has frustrated me or challenged my authority?
3. Have I ever talked "above" or "below" a person's level when I explained things?
4. Do I refer to my patients as parts of the anatomy, e.g., "the back", "the liver", etc.?
5. Do I discuss my patients with other providers in front of them, treating my patients like specimens?
6. Do I try to explain treatment options to my patients and treat them as collaborators rather than children?
7. How would most people rate my bedside manner? Am I distant, close, aloof, caring?

If you are a patient, ask yourself the following questions:

1. Do I treat my doctors as though they were infallible and then get angry when I find out how "human" they are?

2. Do I ask questions if I don't understand?

3. Do I tell my health care providers everything that is important to understand me or do I try my best to put on a good front?

4. Do I see my providers as my partners or my adversaries?

5. Do I play any of the pain games with my providers? When? Which ones?

6. Are there some rewards that I am getting for my pain, such as attention, getting out of unpleasant activities, or others? How can I get those gains directly rather than by being in pain?

Partners, Not Adversaries

If you recognize that you may be contributing to the negative patient-doctor cycle, you will want to do your part to reverse this cycle because it is a no-win situation. The first step for both patients and doctors to recognize is that they need to work in partnership. Both have important information to share about the pain, and only by working together can they get the best results. The pain occurs inside the person, and the patient alone can guide. The provider has special skills and knowledge which he or she can share—as well as the limits of that knowledge.

A few years ago, when one of the authors was having a routine pelvic examination, she thanked her gynecologist afterwards for making her comfortable by telling her exactly what he was doing and helping her relax. He replied, "It is my job to make you comfortable. *If you are not relaxed, I cannot do the examination.*" This illustrates how the patient and doctor need to work in tandem so that the job can be done. In this case, the patient needed to let the doctor know what she required so that he could do his job, and he needed to let her know what was happening so she could relax and do her job. Otherwise, something as simple as a routine examination could not take place.

What does this mean for you if you are a patient? Does being a "good" patient mean one who is submissive, compliant, follows "doctor's orders" blindly without questioning? Is a good patient one who "raises hell" to get what he or she wants? Good patients take active charge of their illness, have an understanding of it and are informed about their pain and their body. In Chapter 4 we talk about that in greater detail. Good patients ask questions and communicate to their providers what they need. They negotiate with their doctors and let them know what has to happen so that they can work together. Although they may be seen as "challenging" and may upset some physicians, most providers would prefer someone who asks specific questions and is actively involved in the program to someone who doesn't say anything and doesn't follow the advice. That does not mean "raising hell" or coming with a hostile, defensive attitude. It just means being assertive and looking after yourself. In the space below, jot down some ways you can be a more active partner in your treatment. You may also wish to ask your providers how you can do that.

_____

_____

_____

_____

_____

_____

_____

_____

_____

_____

If you are a provider, how can you make a patient a partner in your care? "Getting into your patients' shoes" and viewing the world from their perspective is probably the first step. We have been impressed that many of the authors of some of the leading books on pain management have suffered from chronic pain themselves and show an empathy and respect for the patient in their work. Whereas we would not go so far out as to suggest putting yourself in pain, think of how you would like to be treated if you were in pain. Many years ago, on a trip to Canada, we saw this sign which has stood out for us ever since: "It is only the way the cards are being dealt that I am helping instead of being helped." Good doctors should be able to level with their patients and let them know all the facts, even if the facts are "I don't know." Making false assurances and promising cures that don't happen only creates and intensifies the negative cycle. Cheri Register (1987) in her book on living with chronic illness eloquently summarizes what makes a good doctor: "A doctor who is honest about his limits of medical knowledge and who trusts patients enough to make them partners in their care will never summarily dismiss symptoms as imaginary or psychosomatic" (p.220). If you are a provider reading this, jot down below how you could make your patient a more active partner in your care. Better still, ask your patients what you could do to make them more active partners.

_____

_____

_____

_____

_____

_____

_____

_____

_____

_____

It is our hope that patients and their caretakers can work together in win-win solutions rather than spending millions of dollars and emotional energy in this battle which now also involves insurance carriers, attorneys and the courts. Wouldn't it be better if we got out of the blame game, if doctors and patients could say to each other, "Look, we're all trying the best we can. We're frustrated because we can't understand your situation and we'll all try to work together." Maybe then physicians wouldn't need to label and patients wouldn't have an investment in proving that their pain is real. But then, if people knew how to do that, countries wouldn't need to have wars, would they?

A Comprehensive Approach to the Treatment of Chronic Pain

We have so far discussed some of the problems that can occur when looking for a "magic pill" that works for acute pain. If the pain is of a chronic nature, then a comprehensive pain treatment program is needed. Let us look at the components of a multidisciplinary pain program and the principles of chronic pain management.

A chronic pain program should treat the whole person and should take into account physical, mental, emotional, social and spiritual aspects of pain management. Since chronic pain can create so many problems in a person's life, you can not treat the pain by itself but need to address those areas as well.

A chronic pain program is not a short-term "quick fix" but involves a lifestyle change. If pain affects so many areas of life, then pain management must be a way of life. It is not just taking medications but learning to pace and control activities that affect pain.

A pain management program should be individualized and adapted to your unique situation and needs. No two people have the same pain or the same way of handling it. It is important to know you and your situation when making a treatment plan. As William Osler said: "It is much more important to know what sort of patient has a disease than what sort of disease a patient has."

Your treatment program should involve your family. As we shall see in later chapters, you are not the only person whose life has been affected by the pain. Your loved ones need to be educated about pain and the best way of handling it and to be included in most aspects of your program.

A pain management program involves a *team* of professionals who work together and with you to address different aspects of your program. Teams include physicians, psychologists, nurses, social workers, physical and occupational therapists, dieticians and any number of people involved in your feeling better.

Biofeedback

Exercise

Acupuncture

TENS

BEAT CHRONIC PAIN!

Continuing Education

Hypnosis

Relaxation Training

Operant Conditioning

Nutritional Counseling

Individual Counseling   Physical Therapy

Coping Skills Training   Autogenics

Imagery

Nerve Blocks

Your program can include any number of therapies for your pain, such as stress management, biofeedback, medications, physical therapy, nerve blocks, massage, exercise and conditioning, TENS, pain management classes, among other aspects of the program. We will describe some of these treatments in more detail later on in the book.

Summary

In this chapter, we have discussed some of the frustrations experienced by patients when first seeking treatment and look for a "quick fix" which works for acute pain but not for chronic pain. We have outlined some ways for both patients and their health care providers to become partners instead of adversaries. Both patients and their caretakers need to deal with their attitudes before approaching treatment so that it can work. Successful pain management involves a comprehensive multidisciplinary integrated approach.

Chapter 4

Taking Charge

*"The time to fix your roof is before
it starts raining."*

This may be the most important chapter in this book. So far you have learned a great deal about the nature of pain and its treatment. Later on we will teach you more tools for coping with it, but none of the knowledge you have mastered or will acquire can be effective without your active involvement in your healing process. We have spent a great deal of time talking about what can be done *for you* or *to you.* Now we will be talking about what you can do *yourself*—you as a manager. Your physicians and other health providers can only do so much: they can rearrange your muscles and tendons, they can cut and snip, they can try to find the medication that works best for you, they can massage and manipulate your body, they can teach you about the nature of pain and ways to relax it—*but only you can manage your pain.*

"Can anything be done for my pain?" you may ask in frustration. "Why can't anyone help me?" Instead, we encourage you to ask "What can I do about my pain?" because you are the most important person in your care and only you can manage your life and your pain. Within each of us is the power to listen to our pain, understand its signals and turn it off. Within each one of us is the ability to manage our pain.

Management and Managers

So what does the word "manage" mean? Webster's Thesaurus gives numerous synonyms, among them: "to accomplish, administer, arrange, command, control, cope with, deal with, direct, dominate, get along, guide, govern, handle, muddle through, succeed, survive". These words all suggest that we come to terms with pain, either by gaining control over it, getting along with it or only barely surviving it. How well we manage it—whether we succeed or only muddle through it—is what this chapter is about.

Did you ever have to manage a business? A job? A household? Your children? What skills did you use?

_____

_____

_____

_____

_____

_____

_____

_____

_____

_____

As you answered the above questions, you probably recognized that you are using management skills everyday and that you have experience in coping that you can apply to your handling of pain. Some problems are easier to manage than others, of course. It may be simpler to handle your finances if you have lots of money or your kids if they are already well-behaved, just as it may be easier to control your body if you didn't have an injury, but you have to learn to cope within these limitations.

What kind of manager are you? Are you the kind who sets arbitrary rules and demands of your children, employees or yourself and tries to impose them whether they fit or not? Do you seek perfection and then get upset when you can't meet those standards? Do you push your body beyond its limits until it rebels and can't function any longer? Or do you go to the other extreme and ignore the signals from your children, employees or body, letting whatever happens happen, until there is so much chaos and disruption that you cannot ignore it any longer? Are you the kind of manager who goes from crisis to crisis, who puts out one fire after another? Or are you one who plans ahead and prevents disasters before they occur?

So what does good management mean when it relates to your pain? It means knowing your strengths and limits and maximizing them. It means planning ahead to avert problems later on. Good managers have a plan. Good managers also delegate and don't try to do everything themselves. In addition, good managers communicate to others what they are doing. It means learning to manage your pain rather than let it manage you.

John Wayne and Chronic Pain

Every Monday, Phyllis would go to physical therapy for her back, then she would go outside in her yard and mow the lawn. She would mow half the yard, then take her pain medications and complete the job. "After that," she said, "I can't do anything for a week." "And then?" she was asked. "Then my lawn needs mowing again." Phyllis is a good example of someone working against herself without knowing it. Each time she mows the lawn, she reinjures herself and undoes all the benefits she received from her treatment. Why doesn't Phyllis use common sense? Is she stupid? Far from it. She is an intelligent woman who has held responsible jobs, raised lovely children and organized many projects.

Phyllis is typical of many of the people we see with chronic pain: people who have always handled lots of responsibilities,

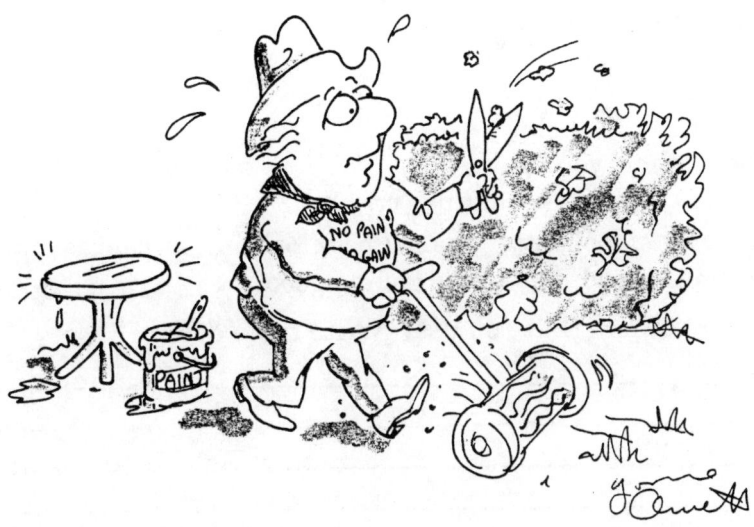

who have been successful all their lives, who have been good providers and parents, people who have pushed themselves to the limit, who were strong and who didn't want to give in to anything—including the pain. John Wayne would have been proud of them! Unlike the stereotype of many patients with chronic pain—that they are "lazy" or that they lie in bed all day—most of the people who come to pain programs are very hard workers and providers. Most have worked long hours, sometimes holding down two jobs. They played hard and parented hard. Sherry, the mother of four, whom we talked about in the first chapter, is a good example ("I used to work two jobs and I used to do things with the kids. I don't mean take them—I mean go *with* them").

People like Phyllis and Sherry have attitudes that reflect the work ethic of America: you keep going until you get the job done, no matter what the cost. They have learned that when you start something, you finish it. They have also learned to be "strong", not to ask for help or to show their pain. They believe that big girls or big boys don't cry, and crying is only for weaklings. They are stoic, and they don't let anybody know what is going on inside. They frequently say, "I'm stubborn", "I won't give in" or "I don't quit".

Below are some of their attitudes about work. Check which of those statements you tell yourself.

- ☐ When you start something, you finish it.
- ☐ No pain—no gain.
- ☐ Push through the pain.
- ☐ Don't stop till you drop.
- ☐ Don't ask for help.
- ☐ Don't show your pain.
- ☐ Don't cry—only weaklings cry.
- ☐ When you feel better, make up for lost time and do as much as you can while you are feeling good.

Are there others that you use? Write them down:

_____

_____

_____

_____

Although there is something admirable about being "strong", "stubborn" and "not a quitter", Phyllis, Sherry and others have used their strength against their bodies. There is a lack of harmony between what they wanted to do and what their bodies were telling them they could. Instead of using their vitality and stubbornness wisely for their benefit, they allow it to deplete them, making their pain worse and laying them up in bed for days. In other words, they let their pain manage them rather than listening to their bodies and have control over it.

Let us take a look at the graph "Monitoring Pain" to see how this works:

15 minutes	➡ A little fatigue *Don't stop*
30 minutes	➡ Much fatigue — Increased pain *Don't Stop*
45 minutes	➡ Exhaustion — Great pain *Don't Stop*
60 minutes	➡ Horrible pain *Don't Stop*
75 minutes	➡ Body about to explode *Stop*

MONITORING PAIN

As you can see from the graph on the previous page, Phyllis and others start an activity, whether it be dusting, typing, or washing the dishes. After roughly fifteen minutes, they start to feel tired. But do they pay attention to their fatigue? Of course not! ("I'm not going to let a little fatigue stop me"). They continue working, and after 30 minutes not only has the fatigue gotten worse but their pain has increased as well. They still keep working because of their attitude that once you start something, you keep going till the job is finished. After 45 minutes, they are exhausted and in great pain but they still don't give in to it. The show must go on—the job must get done, no matter what. After an hour, the pain becomes unbearable, but they still continue to work. After all, they are stubborn and strong and they are not going to let the pain get to them. After 75 minutes, when their body is about to explode, when they can no longer see straight, when they can barely move—then they stop. "Don't Stop Till You Drop!" Unfortunately, they take this expression almost literally and pay a very heavy price for not listening to their bodies at the first stage of fatigue.

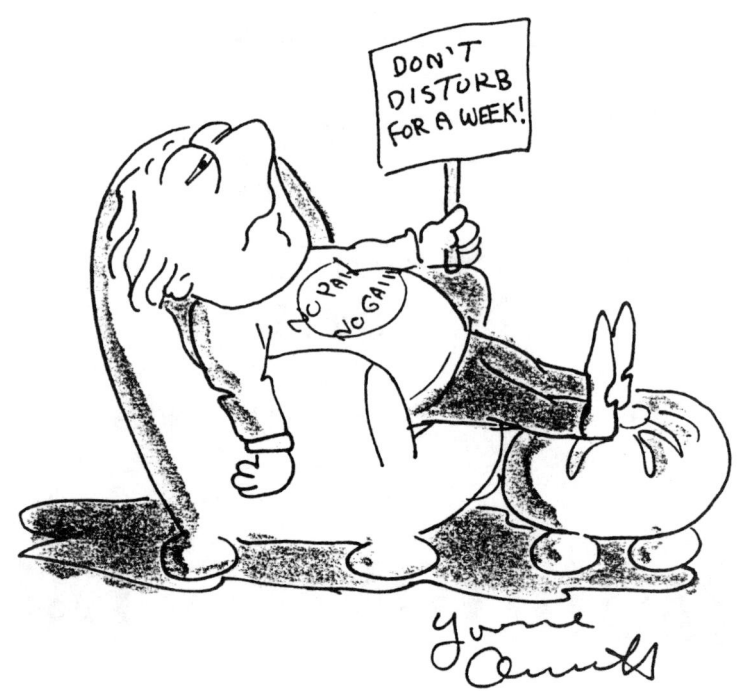

Not only is their failure to listen to their bodies self-defeating because it leads to excruciating pain and being laid up for days, it also results in less being done. Phyllis may spend ten hours doing housework and be worthless for the rest of the week. Or she could pace herself, resting at the first hint of tiredness and maybe accomplishing only two or three hours of housework daily, which is significantly more than the full day of work in the long run—and also more manageable and comfortable!

Typically, many persons with chronic pain have an all-or-nothing work pattern. Like Phyllis who mowed her lawn every Monday after having physical therapy, they tell themselves, "Let me do it while I feel good". They push through the pain ("I'm in charge. I'm not going to give in to it"). Then they drop, and it takes them days to recover. Who is really in charge? Are they taking charge of their pain or are they allowing it to control them?

The next graph shows how this cycle works. As you can see, this is an all-or-nothing pattern. At the first sign of feeling good, they "work till they drop", averaging maybe eight hours of work a week.

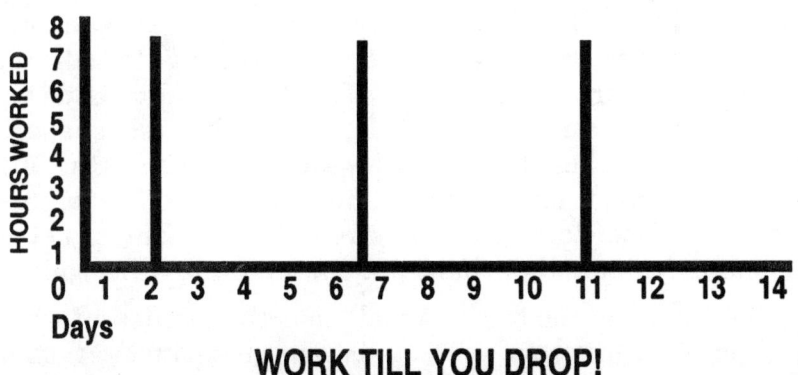

WORK TILL YOU DROP!

Contrast this with the following graph where one takes frequent breaks and works two to three hours a day. This averages to fourteen to twenty-one hours a week, much more than the excruciating eight hours.

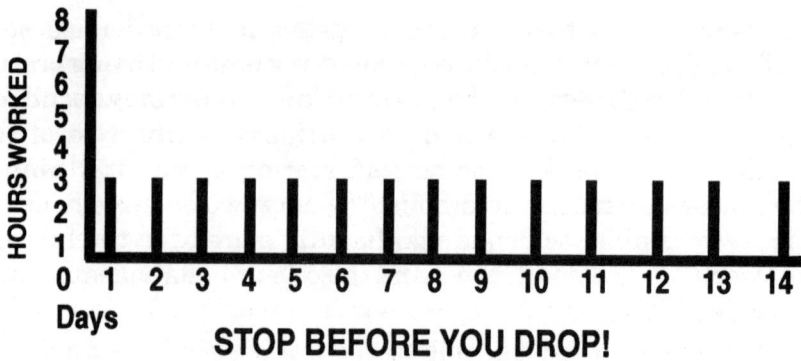

STOP BEFORE YOU DROP!

The most dangerous time for people is when they are feeling good. Maybe you can identify with the feeling of watching all the chores build up and being unable to get to them. You look at the paperwork, at the projects that need completion, at all the things you have wanted to do for so long but couldn't because you were laid up. Now you finally feel good again, and it is *soooo* tempting to push yourself—that's when the disaster happens. If you feel that way, tell yourself to *stop!*

Bill, a man who used to move furniture for a living, talks about his "John Wayne" attitude. "When I first got injured, I kept pushing through the pain and I just stretched and tore my body. But I had to keep working. This was my job. I would work all day long, and then when I got home, I would go to bed—the next day I'd hurt myself again. Thanks to one good doctor finally—he explained to me how I got my body out of shape. I stretched and pulled all my muscles each time. This is the fifth time of building it up—going up and going down. He told me this might be the last time I can stretch it—but I might not go up again. I got another chance—I don't want to do it again.

"I've now learned to stop and do something different when I feel pain—or just stop—period—because the pain I'm getting is just not worth it." How long did it take Bill to learn that? "Three years!" It took the threat of not being able to ever get up again to make him start listening to his body.

Listening to Your Body's Signals

Bill finally learned to develop harmony between his body and his wants. At last he recognized that his body could not take the wear and tear he was imposing on it. "I learned that my body has its own mind. It does what it wants so I am learning not to put it through a lot of stress, and in turn, it stops giving me problems." We have to learn to protect and respect our bodies. Cheri Register compares living with chronic illness to being encased in a portable bubble made of fragile glass. When the body has had a trauma, you have to treat it gently and take care of it. You have to remember that if you have had an injury, your body is damaged and needs your special protection. Many persons with pain can get angry at their bodies and see it as the enemy that refuses to perform. You have to remember that your body is doing its best for you under the circumstances. If you take care of it, it will do more for you, and you will hurt less. If you beat it up and push it around, you will defeat your pain program, create more injury, increase your pain and feel worse. *The choice is up to you.*

Listen to your body and respect it. Listen to your pain. What is it trying to tell you? Rather than ignoring it, get to know it. Ask yourself: Is there a pattern to my pain? Does it occur more at certain times than others? Does it feel better when I sit down, stand up? Is it more pronounced when I'm around certain people? What is it trying to tell me? If you want to feel good, you need a conscious awareness of bodily functions As Cheri Register says, "I wake up in the morning and I test my parts". If you can learn to hear the message your body is telling you, you can adapt your movements to it rather than work against it. We need to be *in harmony rather than in battle* with our bodies.

We need to develop attitudes that are in concert with our body. We have to change our "strong" attitudes that work against us to those that make our pain levels lower. It is very important to keep the pain level low. As we saw, we can accomplish more at a moderate level in one week than do a lot in one day and suffer the negative consequences afterwards. So changing our attitudes can help us in two ways: first, we'll accomplish more; secondly we won't batter our bodies. The self-defeating attitudes that increase pain can be changed to more productive ones. Most important, we need to remind ourselves as Bill did that we may do permanent damage to our bodies for being stoic.

Here are a few attitudes to adopt that keep the pain level lower. Which of these attitudes could you use more of? Check them.

☐ Don't let pain get away from you.

☐ An ounce of prevention is worth a pound of cure.

☐ A stitch in time saves nine.

☐ Nothing is worth it if I'm going to experience pain afterwards.

☐ If I stop now and rest while I'm only a little bit tired, I'll feel better. Afterwards it's too late.

☐ I have to stop it before it gets too bad to control.

☐ Better to do a few things everyday and feel comfortable than to push myself and not be able to do anything afterwards.

☐ The tiredness is a signal that I need to stop.

☐ It's okay to leave early.

☐ It's okay to cut things short.

☐ Maybe I don't have to do this job at all.

☐ If it doesn't get done, it's not the end of the world.

☐ Patience...

☐ One step at a time.

Write down any other attitudes that you can develop to help you monitor your pain.

_____

_____

_____

_____

_____

_____

_____

Tips For Managing Your Pain Before It Manages You

It is not only our attitudes but our work styles that can keep the pain at a lower level. The first of course is: *stop when your fatigue increases and don't let the pain get away from you.* Stop working after only fifteen minutes. If you stop at the first stage of the fatigue level, you don't need to ever get to stage 5. At this level, you can still prevent the pain from getting out of control. At this point, recovery is quick. A nap, relaxation, meditation—all these work: afterwards it may be too late for these methods to be effective. Remember, that's not giving in to the pain—that's preventing your body from being abused.

Another thing you can do is to *break tasks into smaller steps* instead of working until it's all done and you're wiped out. Here are a few suggestions:

* Do a few dishes, rest, then go back and finish.

* Clean one room for the day and not the entire house.

* Let the grocery clerks carry your bags to the car and let someone at home empty them.

* When you ride in a car, get out every hour and take a five minute break.

* Don't sit in one position for more than you can tolerate without taking a break.

Remember, *some tasks are too strenuous and shouldn't be done at all.* Any task that is going to lead to reinjury should be avoided altogether. As Bill told us, "I used to have a lot of junk in the yard that I loved to work on. I made a decision that everything's got to go because I can't do it anymore. So I had the stuff moved out. The less I have to mess with, the better for me." What activities have to be given up of course depend on the nature of the injury but any activity that is going to result in reinjury has got to stop.

Trade off tasks that are too strenuous for you. For example, you can pay the bills while your partner does the laundry. You could do light dusting and let your spouse or children do the heavy vacuuming. You could water the houseplants and hose off the patio and let your family mow the lawn. You could read bedtime stories to the kids or help them with their homework and let your spouse drive them places.

Involve your family in this new approach so that they will understand and have appropriate expectations of you. You must educate your family about what you can or can't do and about the importance of pacing yourself so that you do not experience reinjury. You need to include the family and inform them of what you are doing so they will understand. Otherwise, they will be confused. They will ask you: "You did that yesterday—why can't you do it today?" or "You look well—why can't you do that?" You will need to tell them that the reason you are looking good is because you are taking care of yourself. Involve them in what you are doing. Maybe you can brainstorm together about how you will divide chores. We will talk in more detail about the importance of communicating with your family in a later chapter. A beginning step would be to give your family this chapter to read.

You have to *create a safe environment where you let people know your limitations and learn to say no to activities that will result in reinjury,* such as hiking, going to the zoo, sitting at the movies, shopping for long periods of time or long car trips. It is important that you tell people *in advance* about your need to pace yourself rather than in the middle of an activity to avoid problems later on. For example, if you are planning to go on a long car trip with friends, let them know that you will have to take a break every hour. Tell them "I'm going to have to stop three or four times during the trip. Do you still want to go with me?" They may not or they may say it's okay. That way they can plan on it. If you don't tell them up front, they may get resentful or you may feel guilty and end up doing things that will hurt you later on.

Learn to do activities in ways that don't strain your body. It is important not to put more pressure on your body than is necessary. For example, the type of chair you sit on can be crucial for your comfort level. If your job requires you to sit for long periods of time, get a proper chair. You can also carry a back-ease cushion with you when you go places where there is no comfortable seating.

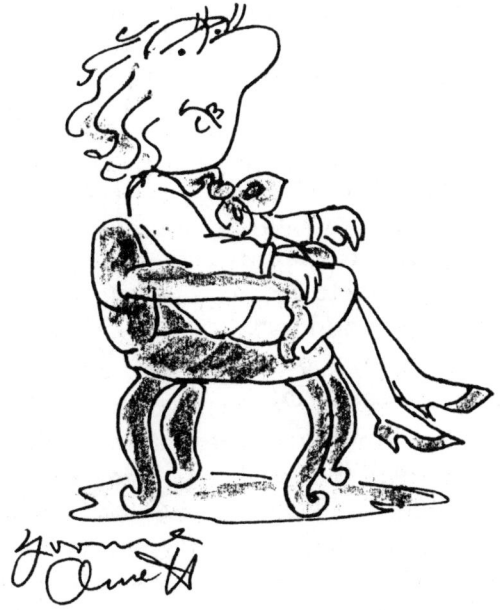

Get a proper chair

Similarly, the type of mattress you sleep on is important. A firm mattress with support or a waveless waterbed will not only put less stress on your back but will help you sleep better. You need to find the appropriate mattress for you. You may need

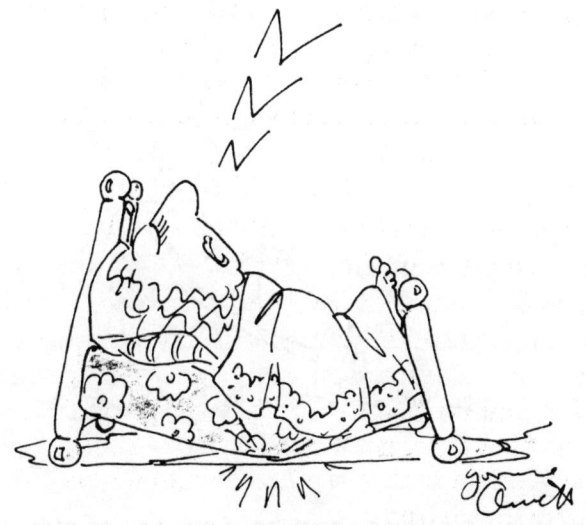

Use a more comfortable mattress.

similar supports for standing. If your job requires you to stand for long periods of time, get a small stool and alternate putting one foot on the stool with another every few minutes. Some people need a cane to support their weight. Don't hesitate to use one if you have to stand for long periods of time. Comfortable shoes are essential, particularly for women who wear high heels that put more tension on the back. Women's handbags can also be a source of strain. Carrying a shoulder bag or tote bag can cause persistent shoulder and backaches. Any bag that weighs over five pounds will do it. If you carry a tote bag, remove as much of the weight from it as you can and try to alternate shoulders. In addition, learn ways of standing, lifting and sitting that will put the least strain on your body. Proper posture is essential, and in a pain program, you can learn correct ways of sitting, standing and lifting that will put the least pressure on your body.

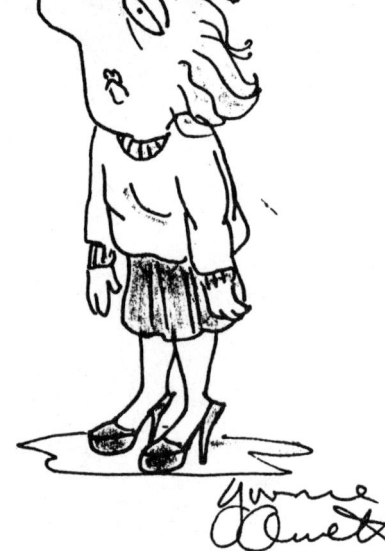

Comfortable shoes are important

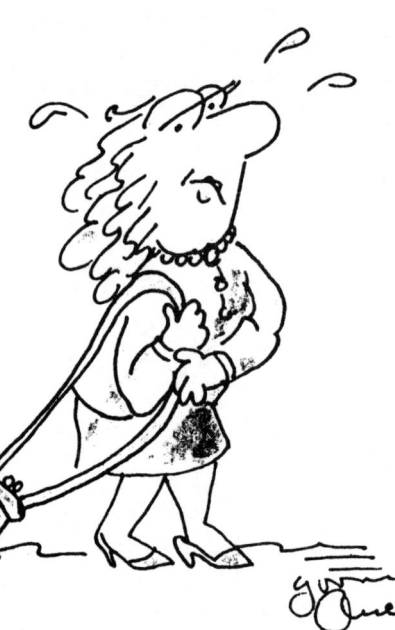

Women's handbags can be a source of strain

Develop a daily routine that helps you and your body rejuvenate. Your routine should include at least three or four half-hour periods to practice some form of relaxation training. It should include adequate sleep, proper nutrition and some type of exercise that has been approved by your physician. It should allow some activity that reduces stress, whether being with friends, listening to music or reading a novel and some time just for "self-indulgence". A daily routine means taking medication on a schedule so that you don't let your pain get away from you. Establishing a liveable routine requires examining which activities you can cut down on and which you may have to give up altogether. It involves setting priorities so that you save your energy for those tasks that are most important.

Maintaining your body has to be your top priority—or you may not have a body to maintain. As Bill said, "I finally realized my priorities. Everything I do, I now try to do with wanting to help me feel better. I may not get a second chance." If managing your pain is your top priority, you have to constantly listen to what your body is telling you and act on its advice. You have to always keep in the back of your mind that staying past bedtime, missing a nap, or overexerting yourself can mean many days in bed afterwards. You must pay attention to when it is your best time and when you are feeling at your worst so you can plan your activities accordingly.

You need to *adopt a way of life that is in harmony with your body's signals.* You have to *rearrange* your life so that you don't have to live with the pain. It's a commitment to yourself to live your life as fully and comfortably as you can and it means adopting habits that let you do so. Knowing that you have limited resources, you have to *plan* in advance how you will approach the day. It requires focusing on *preventing* your pain from getting the better of you in the first place. For example, Bill told us, "I wanted to go to Flagstaff to see the music festival. I went to bed very early the night before so I could get up and go. If I want to do something, I have to plan in advance. I also told myself it's okay to leave early."

Making a commitment to a new way of life is not always easy. It requires a great deal of patience and it means learning that you can't do everything. It may require getting rid of many of the unrealistic standards that we set for ourselves. It also involves learning to deal with the frustrations of not being able to do it all. It means being realistic about our limitations and choosing attitudes and habits that help us manage the pain and learning to live a full life within the reality of our situation.

TIPS FOR PAIN MANAGEMENT

(1) Don't let pain get away from you. Take pain relief at its earliest signs.

(2) Stop and rest. Don't wait till the pain is impossible. Don't "John Wayne" it.

(3 Pace yourself. Break up activities into small steps and do a little at a time, e.g., mow the lawn in 2 or 3 days. The motto, "When you start something, finish it right then", doesn't work for chronic pain.

(4) Learn to relax and practice relaxation 3 or 4 times a day for 1/2 hour each time. Learn biofeedback or medical self-hypnosis or meditation.

(5) If you are on medication, take it at regular times. Don't wait till the pain is impossible. Manage your pain— don't let it get away from you.

(6) Use a TENS unit to block your pain.

(7) Use a back-ease cushion to relieve back strain while sitting.

(8) Learn to do activities in ways which don't strain your body.

(9) Reduce worries, conflicts and physical strains as all these stressors increase your physical pain level.

In the next section, we would like to ask you to look at your life and see what changes you can make to manage the pain before it manages you. You may wish to involve your family in this process. Answer the following questions:

(1) When I start an activity, do I stop to rest after the first sign of fatigue? Do I continue until I am in a little pain? A great deal of pain? Until I am ready to drop? What changes do I need to make?

_____

_____

_____

_____

_____

_____

_____

(2) Which activities or tasks can I break up into small steps?

_____

_____

_____

_____

_____

_____

(3) Which tasks should I give up altogether because they are too strenuous or may cause reinjury?

_____

_____

_____

_____

_____

(4)   Which tasks or activities can I trade off with my family or friends so that I put the least strain on my body?

_____

_____

_____

_____

_____

_____

(5)   How can I involve my family in my new approach? Have I communicated to them about my needs? If not, how can I do so?

_____

_____

_____

_____

_____

_____

(6)   What do I need to tell my friends or co-workers about my need to pace myself? In which situations do I need to be assertive?

_____

_____

_____

_____

_____

_____

(7) What are some modifications I can make to put less stress on my body? Do I need a new chair, a different mattress, a footstool, a smaller handbag, a cane, comfortable shoes? Do I need to stand, walk, lift or sit differently?

_____

_____

_____

_____

_____

_____

_____

_____

_____

(8) What kind of a daily routine can I adopt that will help me? Am I getting enough sleep? Exercise? Am I practicing relaxation four times a day? Does my plan have unstructured time for fun and "self-indulgence"? Am I taking my medications at regular times before the pain becomes impossible?

_____

_____

_____

_____

_____

_____

_____

_____

(9) Am I managing my pain or am I allowing it to manage me? If I choose to manage it, what major adjustments do I have to make? How might I have to rearrange my life? Think very carefully and take a great deal of time to answer this question.

_____

_____

_____

_____

_____

_____

_____

_____

_____

_____

_____

_____

_____

_____

_____

_____

Can you see now why we said that this may be the most important chapter in the book? Or that conscious pain management is a daily event? And that you have to do 90% of the work?

Summary

You can learn to manage your pain or you can let it control you. There are certain attitudes and behaviors that interfere with effective pain management and create a disharmony between mind and body. Learn to listen to your body's signals and pace yourself so you can be an effective manager.

Chapter 5

Emotional Aspects of Pain & Pain Management

"The sorrow which has no vent in tears may make other organs weep."
Henry Maudsley

• Sarah is sitting in her living room watching the evening news. Pictures of war, hunger and violence flash on the screen. Sarah becomes aware of a throbbing pain in her head.

• John is worried about how he will pay the bills this month. He looks at the figures in the checkbook and becomes more and more agitated. He is aware of the sharp pain in his neck.

• Bill starts to discuss his case with his attorney. As he describes his injury and how much it has affected his life, he becomes more and more bitter, and the pain in his back becomes more and more unbearable.

Depression, worry, fear, anger—these emotions can play havoc with our nervous system. They can open up the pain gate, allowing the pain signals to enter. We have already seen how stress can affect how much we hurt. You will remember that soldiers during World War II who had war injuries needed very little medication for their pain compared to civilians with similar injuries. For the soldiers, their wounds meant that they were going home and were not going to die, whereas for the civilians, the injuries made their future uncertain. To the soldiers, their wounds meant less stress, and they hurt less. To the civilians, their wounds meant more stress, and they hurt more. As you can see, there is a powerful two-way interaction between the mind and the body: how we think, feel and behave affects our body, and our physical states can influence our emotions, thoughts and behaviors. More simply put, stress can increase pain, and pain can increase stress. *Anything you can do to lower your stress will lower your pain.*

In this chapter, we will describe the pain-stress cycle in more detail and teach you ways of dealing with your *emotions* to intervene in this cycle. Negative emotions are like sandpaper on the nerves: they open up the pain gate and increase pain levels dramatically. We will talk about anger in much detail because it frequently consumes so much energy and is a toxic drain. Research has found that bitterness and vengeance are the emotional responses most likely to produce high stress levels and affect health. We will also discuss depression, anxiety and other variants of those emotions that are usually subsumed under the category of "stress".

In the next two chapters, we will discuss the effects of our *behavior* and our *thoughts* on our emotions and on our pain levels. Feelings, thoughts and behavior are intricately intertwined, of course, and our separating them into emotional, mental and behavioral aspects of pain is somewhat arbitrary because of the overlap.

The Pain Stress Cycle

The chart on the next page describes in detail how chronic pain and emotional stress interact. As you can see from this diagram, chronic pain frequently leads to reduced ability to function at home or work settings, as it did in Lenny's case. As we have already seen in the first chapter, chronic pain involves lots of *losses*. Persons with chronic pain frequently lose much of their independence and have to depend on others to do what they used to. They are unable to do chores at home or to parent the way they did in the past. They also are unable to do many of the social and recreational activities that gave them pleasure. In addition, the loss of income may often limit their ability for "fun" activities. The ability and desire for sex are also reduced. As we have seen in Lenny's case, this can lead to a host of negative emotions including anger and irritability, guilt, depression and a general lack of energy and enjoyment in

Pain Stress Cycle

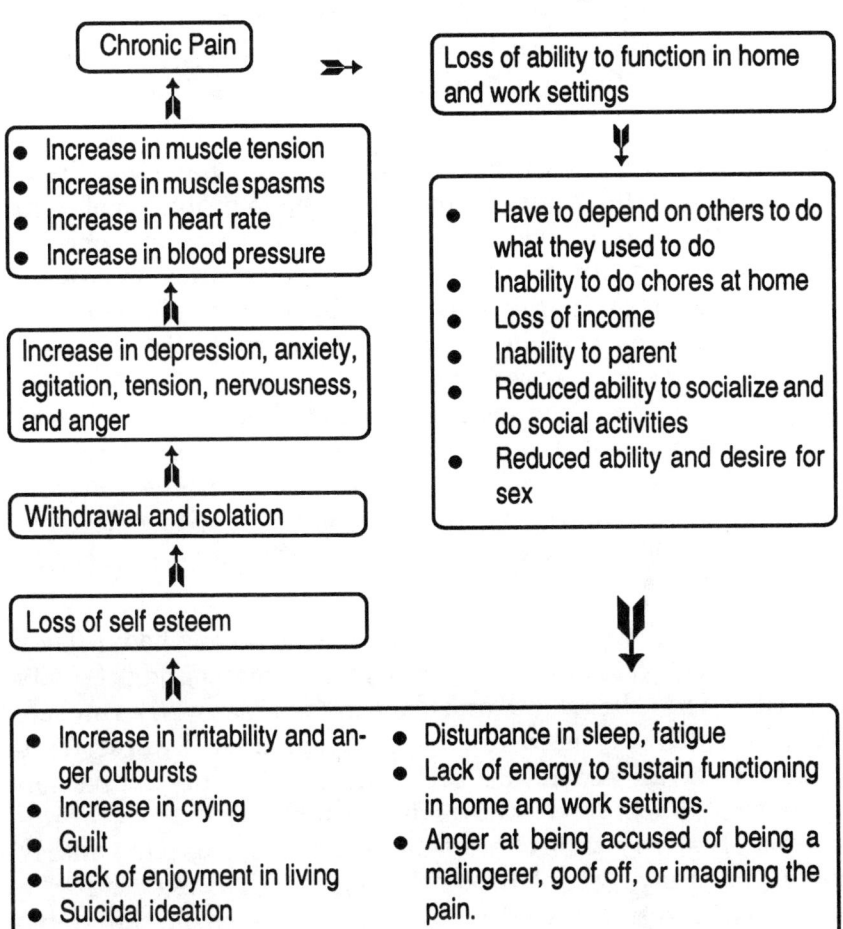

living. This frequently strains their relationships with loved ones, and there is an increase in divorce rates.

Edwina, whose husband left her after many years of marriage, describes the effect all of this had on her self-esteem: "I hate myself for the way things are. Sometimes I can't do anything around the house, it hurts so much. It makes me really depressed at times—most of the time—not only sometimes." The loss of self-esteem as we have seen is tied up to a loss of *identity*. Who am I now that I can't do things around the house, if I can't work, parent, be a provider? There is a lot of emotion connected to the losses because so much of our identity and self esteem is tied up in these roles. So, like Edwina, many people end up hating themselves and feeling that they are worthless.

"I have sisters but they're far away. They have families of their own so I don't upset them. They have problems of their own," Edwina continued. Like her, many persons with chronic pain begin to isolate themselves from others: they don't want to be a burden to their friends or families. This only increases their feelings of worthlessness and depression. We all need people to tell us we are still worthwhile, and it's hard to keep going without a rooting section, without people around us who tell us not to give up hope and that we are still okay. Unfortunately, many persons with chronic pain cut themselves off from the very people who can most provide them with emotional nourishment—which only escalates their feelings of depression and frustration.

These negative feelings are very harsh on the body. They can have a direct impact on our physical organs and intensify muscle tension, heart rate and blood pressure as well as muscle spasms which only aggravate the pain and make it worse. This can become an escalating cycle, with pain and depression reinforcing each other, and both can magnify and spiral upwards. It's easy to get into this negative cycle, particularly when you're laying in bed or not feeling well. To break the cycle and feel better, we need to intervene in each of the steps, including the depression, anger, withdrawal and interactions with others.

It is difficult to state which is the predominant emotion that is associated with pain. Some people emphasize fear or anxiety, others frustration or anger, and others depression, which includes sadness, despair, loneliness, hopelessness, helplessness, anguish and guilt. It can feel like an emotional roller coaster at times when you are having these feelings. Whichever emotion you are experiencing, these feelings can wreak havoc with the nervous system. These emotions have been termed "pain intensifiers" (Brand and Yancey, 1988) because they make the pain so much more unbearable. We will be discussing the emotions of anger, depression and anxiety and what you can do to reduce them.

NEGATIVE EMOTIONS & PAIN

Depression, anger and anxiety are difficult emotions that are like sand paper on the nervous system.

(a) They cause muscles to tighten up and go into spasm.

(b) Tight muscles pull on bones, ligaments, tendons and irritate nerves, increasing pain levels.

(c) Blood vessels contract, resulting in less food and oxygen to the body and less carrying away of waste products.

(d) Reduction in these feelings will benefit you by lowering pain.

(e) Not reducing these feelings can create high strain on the body that decreases or stops the benefit of treatment from your doctors and physical therapists.

(f) Anything you can do to cut down negative emotions will make your pain less and your treatments more effective.

Healthy and Unhealthy Anger

Anger is one of the most difficult and misunderstood emotions. It is a healthy, normal and real emotion and is a natural reaction to loss. If you recall the "Good Grief" cycle, anger is one of the stages that needs to be dealt with to resolve the identity crisis. It is important to know how to cope with anger because not expressing it properly can affect your health. A growing body of literature reflects on the negative effects of anger and hostility on your health:

- A 12 year longitudinal study of 10,000 people revealed that those who *suppressed* anger were more than twice as likely to have died of heart disease as those who openly expressed anger.

- A 25 year study showed that people with high *hostility* scores had higher incidence of heart disease; they were also six times more likely to die by the age of fifty from *all* causes of disease than their lower-scoring controls.

What do these contradictory studies tell us? Is it better to suppress anger or to be openly hostile? Neither is good for your health. Anger needs to be expressed rather than stifled, but hostility and anger are not the same. Healthy anger is speaking up assertively and expressing your needs in a direct manner. Unhealthy anger can be either "stuffing your feelings" or expressing them indirectly by withdrawal, coldness, resentment or sarcasm. It may also mean taking your frustrations out on others rather than at what is really bothering you. The most destructive anger for our health is hostility: the hate, resentment and bitterness that fester inside us and that grind at our internal organs.

If you have anger, you must deal with it: it will not go away on its own. If it is not addressed, it will release its poison in the body and affect healing. However, if you continue to focus on it and hold on to the bitterness and resentment, it will have a vicious effect on your health. Joan Borysenko* (1994) calls this type of anger "marinated toxic waste" where we can stew in our own juices till the anger engulfs us and pervades our bodies and our lives.

What are some healthy ways to express anger? The first step of course is to *recognize that you are angry and choose what to do about it.* You need to be able to express it and let it out. If you are angry at someone, speak up about the situation and try to do it in a manner that is respectful to you and that person. Using "I" language is important because it doesn't attack. "I feel irritated that you didn't show up" is preferable to a "you" statement such as "*You* are so irresponsible", which can only intensify the hostility. When you have a gripe with someone, it is better to get it off your chest than to let it fester.

If there is no proper outlet for the anger, you may still need to let it out in other ways so that it doesn't remain in your body. Writing down your feelings in a journal can help you release

---

*Workshop conducted in Phoenix, Arizona in October 1994.

them. Talking to a trusted friend, spouse or therapist about your frustrations can also be very useful. Everybody needs a place where they can say "This sucks". Crying is a very healthy outlet and may help release some of the tension in your body. Physical outlets are also very good for anger, whether it be beating on a punching bag or screaming at the top of your voice when nobody is around. The idea is to *let the tension out rather than hold it in.* The point of all of these outlets is *release and relief.*

But be careful here. If it is an old issue and you keep *rehashing* it, then it provides no physical or emotional release and only increases the tension in your body. This is the type of anger that you "marinate" in and allow to poison you. This is the type of anger that festers inside you, and each time you bring it up, increases your negative emotions until you are wallowing up in it. This is the anger from the past that you have talked about and cried about and can no longer do anything about, the kind of anger that hurts nobody else but you. Many persons with chronic pain are so focused on how they have been wronged that they let it consume every aspect of their lives. True, they have a right to their anger and the whole injustice of their situation. However, *wallowing in those negative emotions only hurts them.*

Nathan put it this way: "One night when I was tossing and turning and unable to sleep because I kept going over and over what that s.o.b. had done to me, it suddenly occurred to me that I am the one who is staying awake hurting. He's not hurting. He's probably sleeping peacefully. If I let go of my anger, I'm the one who will benefit. I'm not getting to him at all. *I need to let go for me.*" Nathan has decided that he would stay away from situations which he called "bitch sessions", and he would stop complaining and indulging in negativity because that only fans the flames. "When I have these thoughts now, I can make them worse or I can say, "It's over and done with and I want to go on with my life. There's no profit in it for me." This is of course easier said than done, and letting go is not so simple. We will be talking about some ways of doing that.

The following table summarizes the differences between healthy and unhealthy anger:

HEALTHY & UNHEALTHY ANGER

ANGER THAT HEALS	ANGER THAT HURTS
■ Serves as a release	■ Festers and smolders
■ Is communicated openly	■ Is communicated indirectly by emotional withdrawal, coldness, resentment, bitterness, sarcasm, put-downs
■ Is expressed directly	■ Is taken out on self or others
■ Attacks the issue	■ Attacks the person
■ Is expressed in "I" language	■ Is expressed in "You" language
■ Reduces tension and pain	■ Increases tension and pain

What are some ways of getting rid of unhealthy hostility? "I have a *choice,* daily, regardless of how I feel, I have a choice to forgive or to continue to stew about it. I'm learning on a day to day basis that I have a choice to forgive or to continue hating. *Not because I feel like it* but I choose to forgive because it's not doing anything for me", said Dora, a woman who had countless tragedies in her life. "I see a lot of people whose bodies are better then mine but their minds are hurting."

Like Dora and Nathan, there are some statements we can tell ourselves that reduce our anger and there are others that provoke us further and fan the flames. The table on the next page shows us some anger-provoking versus anger reducing thoughts.

Not only do we need to change our thoughts to reduce anger, it is also important to alter our behavior. One of the most destructive ways to fan the flame of hate is in long and bitter discussions of how you were wronged. This is very tempting to do but all it does is have deleterious effects on your body. We will discuss pain talk in more detail later on. If there is a discussion already going on, try to change the subject. If you

ANGER-PROVOKING THOUGHTS	ANGER REDUCING THOUGHTS
OUT OF CONTROL ■ "Why is this happening to me?"	**IN CONTROL** ■ "What can I do about this situation?"
SELF-BLAMING ■ "It's all my fault"	**SELF-BOOSTING** ■ "I'm doing the best I can"
HIGH EXPECTATIONS ■ "It's not fair!" ■ "This shouldn't have happened"	**REALISTIC EXPECTATIONS** ■ "Life isn't fair. I just have to do the best I can under the circumstances."
FOCUSING ON THE PAST ■ "I will never forgive or forget what has happened"	**STAYING IN THE PRESENT** ■ "I'm the only one who is hurting from this" ■ "I choose to reduce my anger rather than let it hurt me" ■ "I'm the one who will benefit" ■ "It's over and done with and I have to go on with my life" ■ "Don't throw good money after bad" ■ "Talking about it will only fan the flames and make me feel worse" ■ "It is easier to love than to hate"

can't, tell people it only hurts you more if you get bitter, or in extreme cases — *leave*. The negativity is not good for you, and you don't want to pick up other people's negative energy. You of course have a great deal of control about these discussions and don't need to start them yourself. Instead, choose to focus on positive events and activities that bring you pleasure. Music, relaxation, artwork, beauty—all of these relax you. Negative thoughts make you hurt.

What Can I Do About My Anger?

Now that we have looked at healthy and unhealthy ways of expressing your anger, let us look at ways of recognizing and dealing with your own anger. Look at the following illustration and see which of these sources of anger you can identify with.

WHERE DOES ANGER COME FROM?

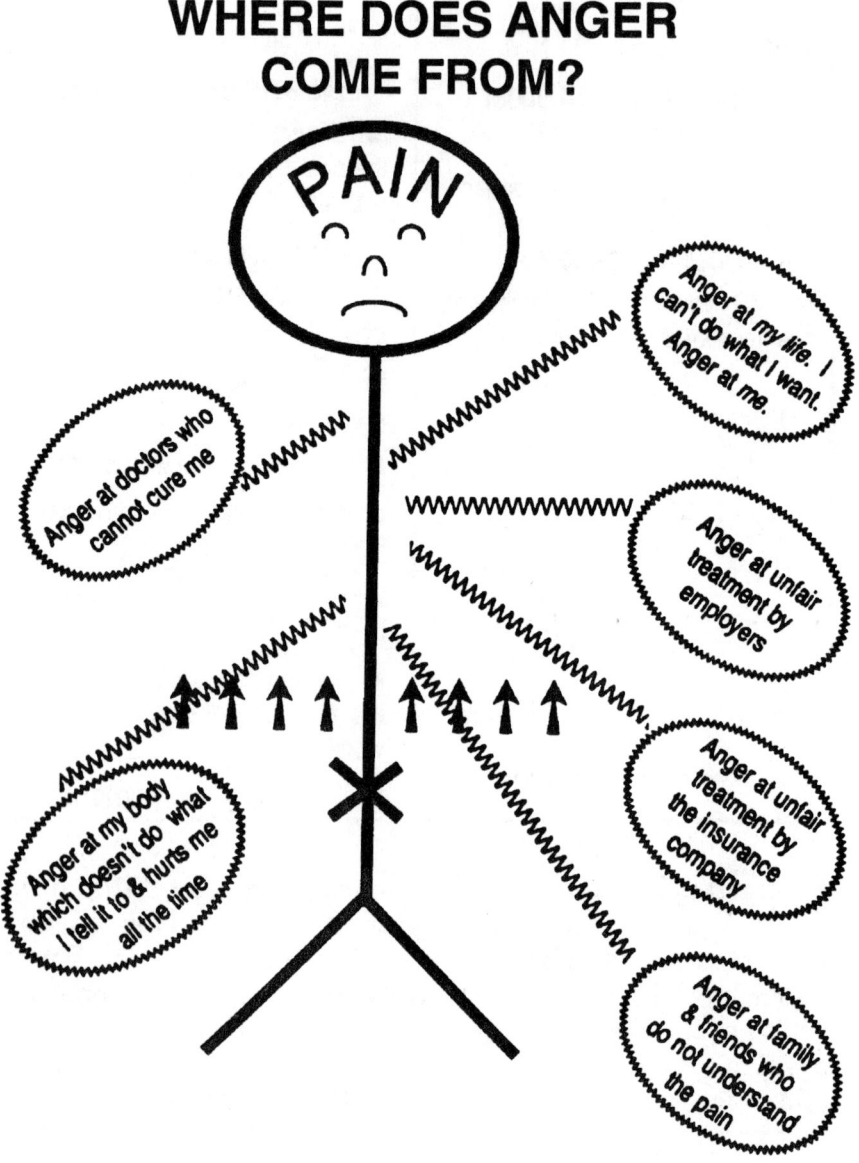

Whom am I angry with?

Place a check mark by any of these that apply and add others that are not covered here.

☐ Boss

☐ Insurance Company

☐ Doctors

☐ Lawyers

☐ Spouse

☐ Children

☐ Other family members

☐ Friends

☐ My Body

☐ Myself

☐ Life

Others:

_____

_____

_____

_____

_____

_____

_____

_____

_____

_____

I can reduce my anger with these people by:

Boss _____

Insurance Company _____

Doctors _____

Lawyers _____

Spouse _____

Children _____

Other family members _____

Friends _____

My Body _____

Myself _____

Life _____

Others

_____

_____

_____

_____

_____

_____

_____

_____

_____

_____

_____

_____

_____

_____

_____

_____

Anger Reduction

(1) If it can be dealt with—reduce it.

(2) If it is in the past and done with—let go of it.

(3) You have a right to be angry, but anger of the past only hurts you.

Remind yourself: If it is in the past, your anger only hurts you. When you can't sleep at night with anger—only you are being hurt.

Anything you can do to *let go* of the anger *will help you* feel less pain.

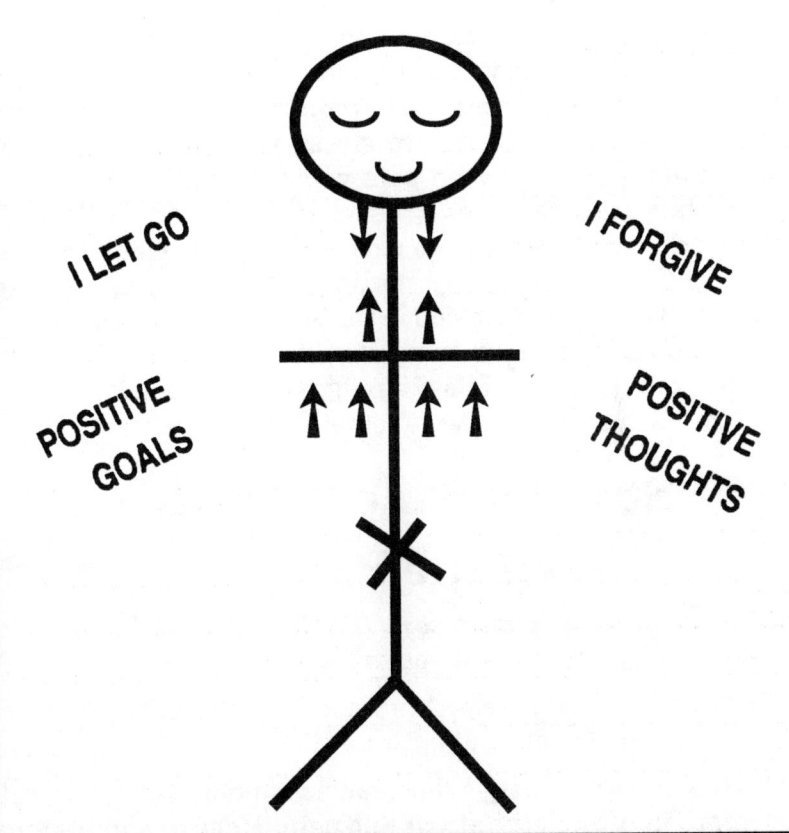

The Pain Drain: Depression, Anxiety & Other Emotions

Depression is an emotion that encompasses so many words: sadness, melancholy, lack of pleasure. It involves guilt, self-hate, feelings of worthlessness, loneliness. When we are depressed, we withdraw and intensify these feelings even more. We feel fatigued, worthless, drained of energy. We feel hopeless and helpless and may even wonder why we need to go on. Anxiety and fear are also a part of this emotional picture. We worry about what's going to happen, we are afraid, we feel so nervous and tense, we don't know what to do. We don't need to describe this emotional roller-coaster to you: these feelings usually go under the general heading of "stress".

What we want to do most of all is help you realize the negative impact these hard emotions have on your body and teach you some ways to reduce them. As we said before, all these emotions are pain intensifiers and only worsen your pain. They allow the gate to open and the pain to be felt more strongly. Anything you can do to reduce stress will lower your pain. Whereas many persons with pain will not go see a counselor because they are afraid that it will confirm that "it *really is* all in my head", we encourage you to do so if you are feeling any of these emotions. Everybody needs a safe place to express feelings and reduce the tension in the body. Support groups are also excellent if they don't turn into "bitch sessions" that only intensify your pain. The following suggestions are not meant in lieu of counseling but are ways to help you feel better.

Staying Sane In Spite of the Pain

1. *Get enough sleep and rest.* Establish a regular time to take a daily nap, even if you are working.

2. *Get regular exercise* within your physical limits. Relaxed muscles lead to relaxed nerves.

3. *Listen to your body.* When you are under stress, you get symptoms of anxiety, fatigue and pain. Heed its signals and

back off. Live in harmony with your body's limitations, and it will do its best for you.

4. *Avoid hurry, flurry and worry.* Pace yourself and lower your standards. Some things can get done tomorrow; some things don't need to be done at all.

5. *Use relaxation at regular intervals* four times a day: when you wake up, around noon, in the late afternoon and before bedtime.

6. *Establish a regular routine* and stick to it. Make sure this includes sleeping, eating and relaxing.

7. *Have something to look forward to each day* whether it's reading a magazine, meeting a friend or working on a project.

8. *Take time each day with your personal appearance.* Buy yourself some things that will help you look and feel better.

9. *Identify your fears.* It might be helpful to write them down and discuss with family, friends or your therapist. Educate yourself about the things you are afraid of. Learn about your pain and treatment and how you can be an active participant.

10. *Avoid self-pity.* It is a waste of time and energy, a "pain drain". Although it is normal to have periods of "Why me?", don't wallow in it.

11. *Try to laugh more.* Laughter is a good tension breaker. Attempt to put some humor in your life on a daily basis.

12. *Love more.* The more love and caring you can give to yourself and others, the better you will feel.

13. *Avoid loneliness.* Even if you feel like withdrawing, remind yourself that getting involved with others helps you feel better.

14. *Avoid self-blame and guilt.* These emotions help no one and only make you feel worse.

15. *Pay attention to your thoughts and change the destructive ones to positive ones.*

16. *Communicate with the people you love and let them know what your needs are.*

17. *Do some volunteer work* if you are unable to work full-time.

18. *Remind yourself that you are in control, and that whereas you cannot control many situations or people, you have control in how you deal with them.*

19. *Add some healthy pleasure to your life.* This last point is so important that we want you to spend time elaborating on it.

Which of these suggestions will you be putting to use? Write them down.

_____

_____

_____

_____

_____

_____

_____

_____

_____

_____

_____

_____

_____

_____

_____

_____

_____

_____

Healthy Pleasures

Research has shown that feeling good is good for your health and that many people are not getting their minimum daily requirement of sensual pleasure (Ornstein and Sobel, 1989). Fortunately for us, we have a pleasure machine inside our head, and our brains have the capacity to produce their own morphine-like substances to make us feel calm. What scientists have found is that the areas of the brain that control emotion are particularly rich in receptors for those chemicals. Researchers have also found that the healthiest, most robust people *expect pleasure in much of what they do.* What distinguishes healthy from unhealthy people is primarily in how much pleasure they put into their lives. When we feel pleasure—after a good nap, a delicious meal or a watching the sunset—these pleasant sensations travel to the brain and make use feel even better. What does this mean for you? If you want to feel good—physically and emotionally—you need to increase the simple pleasures in your life.

We need to think of ways to increase pleasures across all the senses—*sight, touch, hearing, taste,* and *smell.* Touch is one of the most important senses. In one study, a group of patients with chronic muscle tension, body aches and pain got massage treatment for ten sessions. Although these people had not responded to other treatment, most reported less tension, pain and need for medication. Hugs, massages, stroking—these are so vital for us. In a later chapter, we will talk about sexual pleasures as well as part of healing. Many people forego that part of their life altogether which deprives them of one of its most satisfying pleasures.

Heat is also very important to experiencing pleasure. Most of us seek out sunny climates and gravitate towards warm spots. Saunas, steam baths, and hot tubs are not only relaxing, they also reduce muscle and joint pain. In one study, it was found that sitting in a sauna for 30 minutes increased blood levels of beta-endorphins, the internally produced chemicals that relieve pain and produce a "high".

Sight is another sense that is very significant. For example, looking at natural landscapes can produce feelings of friendship, love and calmness compared with urban sights that produce more stress. Try to surround yourself with natural beauty and have positive images in your mind.

Music also "soothes the soul" and can produce feelings of euphoria. Music therapy is useful in the treatment of many illnesses, including headaches, depression and anxiety. Taste and smell are other senses to attend to. Who has not had the experience of feeling deliciously satiated after a mouth-watering meal? To eat slowly, to savor every bit, to enjoy the flavor— that can be one of life's simplest delights. Scent has been one of the most ignored of the human senses, but pleasing smells, because of their connection with the brain's emotion-producing areas, have a great subconscious influence on our moods and memories. Aromatherapy has been used to treat insomnia, anxiety, back pain and migraines. Some people with chronic pain are taught muscle relaxation while inhaling peach fragrance. Later they simply take a whiff of the peach and feel relaxed.

Movement can also bring on blissful feelings. It doesn't only heal but makes one feel good. Exercise releases those pleasure-producing chemicals. Naps are probably one of life's most simple and forgotten pleasures. They can refresh: clearing the mind, relaxing the body and feeling less fatigued. Happiness consists of these simple delights rather than winning the lottery or going to Europe.

Are you getting your daily quota of healthy pleasures? In the space below, write down all of the simple joys you could add to your life, using each of the senses.

Sight:

_____

_____

_____

_____

_____

Touch:

_____

_____

_____

_____

_____

Hearing:

_____

_____

_____

_____

Taste:

_____

_____

_____

_____

Smell:

_____

_____

_____

_____

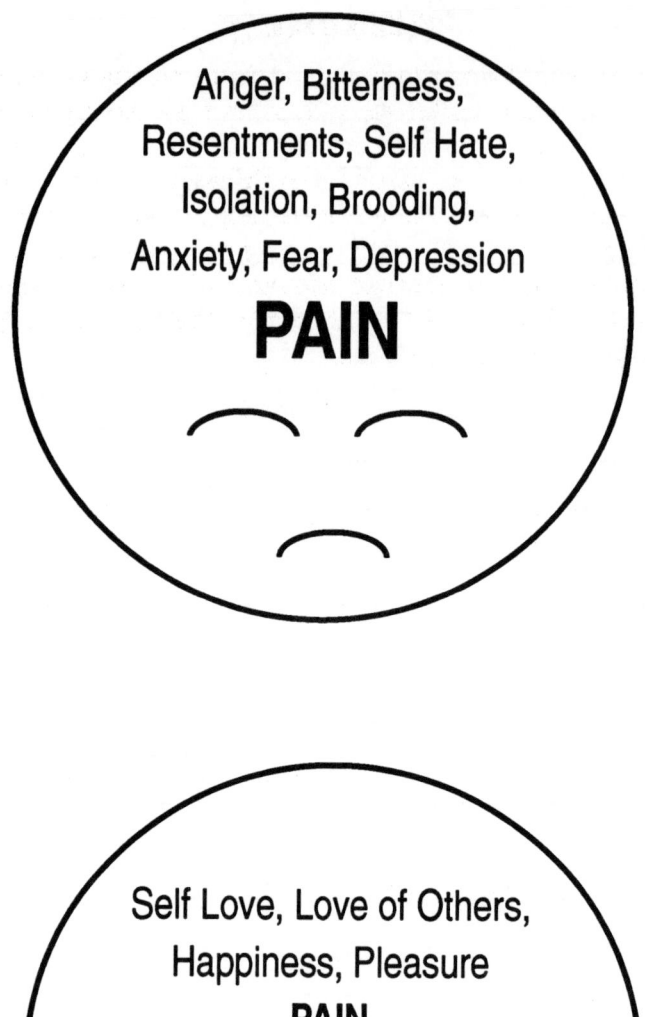

Summary

Negative emotions are like sandpaper on the nervous system. They cause muscles to tighten and go into spasms, and they open the pain gate, making the pain worse and decreasing the benefits of your treatment. Anything you can do to reduce negative emotions will make your pain less and your treatment more effective. Rather than festering in these toxic emotions which only drain you, concentrate instead on increasing pleasure in your life because that increases the brain's morphine-like substances that reduce the pain.

Chapter 6

Behavioral Aspects of Pain & Pain Management

"If a man thinks about his physical and moral state, he usually discovers that he is ill."
Goethe

Don't Groan So Loud: Your Pain Nerves Are Listening!

We have talked about how our *emotions* affect pain and have given you some suggestions for dealing with these hard emotions so they don't make your pain worse. We would like to describe specific *behaviors* that also aggravate the pain. Some pain specialists talk about a pain life-style which may be very hard to give up. Many persons with pain may unconsciously be doing things as grimacing, moaning, wincing, rubbing their temples and in every way calling attention to their pain. Other pain behaviors include sighing, "suffering in silence", asking others to adjust their pillows or fetch them things they can do themselves. Pain behavior also includes constantly talking about pain and switching the conversation to it. Frequently asking for medications is another pain behavior.

The main reason not to talk about pain is that it will make you feel better. "I went to a party one night", John told us, "and after a half hour the hostess came up to me and said she was amazed that I was sitting there all this time without feeling any pain. As soon as she said that, I started to hurt. I couldn't believe that all it took was for her to make one comment about my pain to start to feel it again!" When someone asks you how you are feeling, you immediately start to scan your nervous system and open up the pain pathways which only amplifies the pain. You need to move your attention away from the pain sites or it will make your pain worse. As much as you possibly can, try to not talk about your pain: it's just not good for you.

PAIN TALK & PAIN

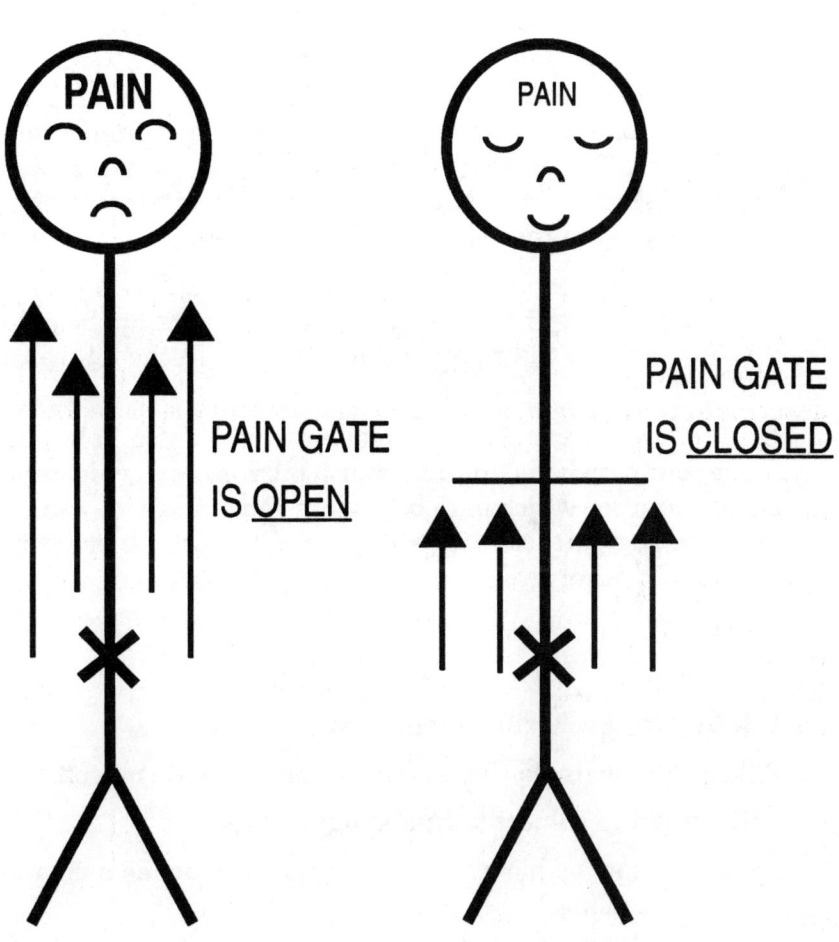

In some treatment centers, they give patients mirrors to see if they are engaging in pain behaviors. Sometimes patients are asked to observe other patients to see if they can see themselves in them. This has two purposes: to see how it feels to be around people who exhibit pain behaviors and to see if you have them yourself.

When persons can see pain behaviors in other people, they can see what their behavior looks like and feels like to other people. Pain behavior is very uncomfortable for others and frequently a *turn-off.* When people complain about their pain, it alienates others and they want to withdraw. Instead of getting compassion or sympathy, it elicits discomfort from others so that they can hardly wait to get away or it may result in some unwanted advice, as it did for Jane who constantly talked about her pain and how much worse it was getting. This brought on numerous suggestions from her friends, family and doctors about different treatment options which only succeeded in infuriating her. Jane did not realize that it was her own pain behavior that led to these "helpful" suggestions.

Secondly, pain behavior increases your pain. When people look inside to see how they are feeling, they will open up the pain tracks and increase their pain, as you can see in the figure on page 85.

The following are some things you could do to help you decrease your pain behaviors. Look in a mirror or at a videotape of yourself and see which pain behaviors you engage in. Which of the following pain behaviors do I show? Check those that apply and add others:

☐ Moaning

☐ Grimacing

☐ Holding my back, rubbing my temples, etc.

☐ Asking people to do things for me that I can do myself

☐ Changing the subject to talk about my pain

☐ Giving a blow by blow description when someone asks me how I am feeling

☐ Asking for medications

Other:

_____

_____

_____

_____

_____

_____

_____

_____

_____

_____

_____

Ask your family and friends which of these behaviors you display. Write those down.

_____

_____

_____

_____

_____

_____

_____

_____

_____

_____

_____

Tell your family and friends (particularly your children who are good observers) to give you a signal whenever you engage in these behaviors.

Observe other people who show pain behaviors. What feelings does that bring up in you? It may be uncomfortable to see yourself in others if you are engaging in unnecessary pain behavior, but this may be a strong incentive to reduce these behaviors only *because they make you hurt more.*

Remember the main reason not to engage in pain behavior is you will feel better!

Don't Ask Me How I'm Feeling: My Pain Nerves Can Hear You!

Ask the people you know well not to ask you about your pain. Your friends and family will naturally ask about your health to show their concern. You need to educate them that this only makes you feel worse. Tell your friends and family: "Don't ask me how I feel. Just say hi, nice to see you." For others, whom you don't know well, remember, that "how are you" is only a greeting and just say "fine" and change the subject. *The whole reason for not talking about pain is you will feel better.*

There is a time to talk about pain, and that is in terms of your limitations. In previous chapters, we asked you to educate your friends and family about what you can or can't do, but they frequently will forget and ask you to go camping, fishing or the movies. You will need to frequently re-educate them because they may get confused. They will say, "You look fine" or "Come on, you can do that" or "Please, we really want you to join us." What they are saying is that they want to be with you. You need to be the best judge of what you can or can't do. You might be able to compromise, as one woman did when her husband wanted her to go play bingo with him. They took two cars, and she left early. So if you can't do a full activity with your family or friends, do part of it. For example, they could go to the movies without you if you can't sit for two hours but you can have dinner together afterwards. Remember, when you talk about pain, only do so to educate.

WHEN TO TALK ABOUT PAIN

Talking about pain opens up pain tracks and increases pain.

1. When people greet you and ask you how you are feeling, say fine and change the subject.

2. Teach family and friends not to ask about the pain and pain problems.

Talk about pain only to educate and prevent reinjury.

1. Tell your family what your limits are. Do it once, teach them and get off the subject of focusing on pain.

2. Don't talk about your pain, except to your doctor to provide information.

The benefits are:

LESS PAIN FOR YOU!

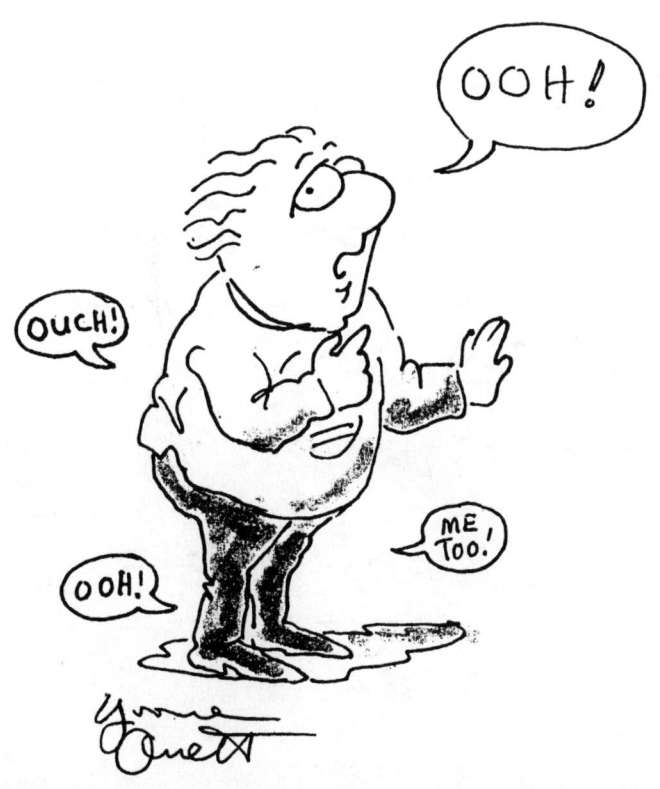

Laugh And Your Pain Nerves Will Laugh With You

Laughter is said to be the best medicine, and we encourage it as an alternate behavior to pain talk. Many persons with chronic pain have lost their sense of humor and find little to smile about when they are not feeling well. However, a hearty laugh can have a direct physiological effect on the body and can make a person feel both physically and emotionally better. Norman Cousins (1976) writes about the curative effects of laughter on his illness: "I made the joyous discovery that ten minutes of genuine belly laughter had an anesthetic effect and would give me at least two hours of pain-free sleep." Laughter as a pain killer? You bet!

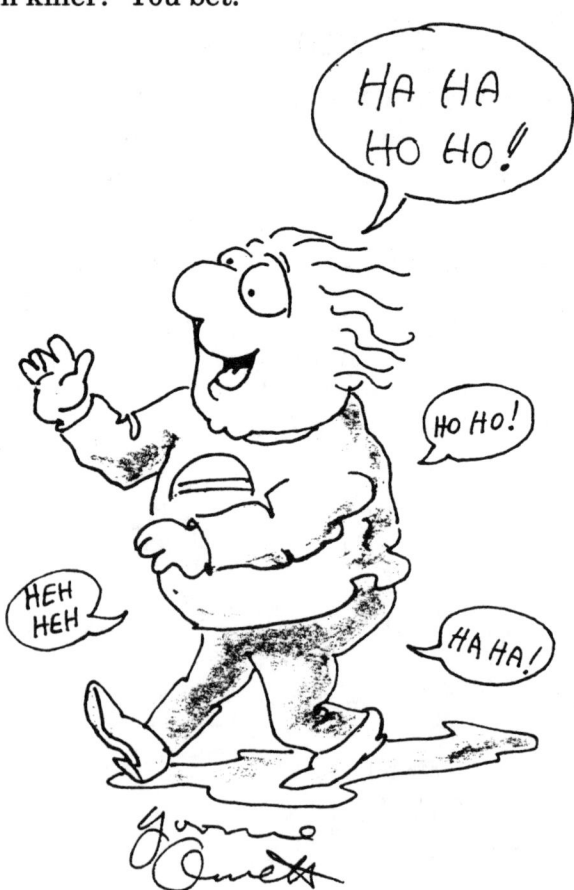

Laughter can clear the respiratory system, reduce tension and provide healthy emotional release. Laughter can close the pain gate and not let the signals through. As Bill told us: "It's hard when things walk away from you that you've had all your life. The most important thing you have is yourself and the most you can do is take care of yourself. Sometimes I look at myself in the mirror and say, 'Well, you don't look in that bad a shape' and then I laugh. I try to keep my sense of humor. I poke fun at everything. And you know what? Then it doesn't seem so bad. I feel much better." So the next time you are feeling down, try to see the funny side of things instead!

Summary

Pain talk and pain behaviors increase your pain levels because when you think about pain, you start to scan your nervous system and open up the pain pathways.

Remember:

When I complain, it increases the pain.

Tell your family:

"Don't ask me how I'm feeling. My pain nerves can hear you!"

Instead of pain talk, adopt laughter as a pain behavior.

Chapter 7

Mental Aspects of Pain & Pain Management

"What takes place in a person's mind is the most important aspect of pain—and the most difficult to treat or even comprehend. If we can learn to handle pain at this third stage, we will most likely succeed in keeping pain in its proper place, as servant and not master."

Paul Brand, M.D. & Philip Yancey,
Pain: The Gift Nobody Wants

How can we use our mental resources as an ally rather than as an enemy to manage our pain and not let it turn into suffering? We can employ our mind to help us in all three stages of the pain cycle: signal, message and response. Our perception of the pain can alter whether our pain signals communicate a message to the brain and how the brain in turn responds to the pain. In other words, we can use our vast mental capacities to keep us from feeling the pain and also from turning it into misery.

There is a large body of scientific literature which shows that our thoughts, beliefs and perceptions about illness influence how we respond to it. We can learn to form attitudes that help us master the pain and to prevent it from turning into suffering. We would like to share with you some of these findings so that you can use them to help you in all of the stages of the pain cycle.

We will first describe some methods which intervene in the first stage of the pain cycle: various forms of relaxation and imagery techniques that can decrease the pain signals and lower the pain. Secondly, we will talk about attitudes and beliefs that make us more vulnerable to pain and illness in general and how we can change those. We will also discuss how we can learn to perceive pain and ourselves as persons with pain in a different way so that it doesn't negatively color every area of our lives.

Learning Relaxation & Visualization Techniques to Reduce Pain

How can we use our mind power to lower our pain? You may be thinking that pain is pain, and it makes no difference what your mind says about it. That's not true. How you experience the pain depends a great deal on what is happening in your mind. Let us take two men who are in a dentist's office, both going to have minor gum surgery. Don has been upset for many days, anticipating terrible pain just like he had experienced the last time he went to the dentist. As he drives to the dentist's office and thinks about what is going to happen, he becomes more and more nervous. While in the dentist's chair, he notices everything the dentist is doing and feels anxious before the dentist even begins the procedure. As you might well have guessed, he has a horrible experience and feels the pain in spite of the novocaine.

Jerry, on the other hand, has a very different kind of experience. He doesn't anticipate any problems, and going to the dentist for him is just another chore he has to do during the day. He also has learned some relaxation techniques to use while in the dentist's chair and utilizes that time to travel in his mind to Europe and revisit all of the beautiful sites he had seen.

Sometimes he would try a different visualization: "I'd picture the pain as little bubbles, and I would blow them out of my consciousness, one at a time, until they all disappeared. At other times, I simply transfer all of that discomfort to my little finger."

Is Jerry using magic? Of course not. He is simply employing some fairly simple relaxation and visualization techniques to help him lower his pain level. There are a number of methods that have been used very successfully to prevent and alleviate pain, including deep muscle relaxation, meditation, autogenics, biofeedback and hypnosis. Many of these processes combine imagery to make pain reduction more effective. The fact that pain is a learned sensation that is mediated in the mind makes it particularly responsive to the effects of visualization.

We will describe the different methods, but only you can determine which one will work best for you. Regardless of which one you prefer, there are a few things for you to keep in mind. First, a word of caution: *these are all learned techniques, and they take lots of practice.* Many people use some of these procedures a few times and get discouraged when they feel no difference in their pain levels right away. It has been our experience in pain programs that *IT WILL TAKE AT LEAST TWO WEEKS OF HALF HOUR PRACTICE SESSIONS FOUR TIMES A DAY TO START FEELING THE EFFECTS.* Many people will not start getting the benefits until after 60 or 70 practice sessions—which means between two to three weeks of continued practice.

Secondly, we strongly recommend *learning these techniques with a therapist* at the beginning and later practicing on your own. Many people are unable to learn to relax just from a relaxation tape or from meditating on their own. A therapist trained in these methods can help you find the best way to relax and the imagery that fits best for you. Your therapist can also make a tape for you to use on your own.

Thirdly, we encourage you to *learn these techniques when your pain level is manageable* and not when it is so high that you cannot concentrate. Remember, you want to use these techniques to lower your pain and to prevent it from getting worse. As we said before, the best time to fix your roof is not when it's raining.

Fourth, once you learn these techniques and get benefits from them, continue to use them on a daily basis. You need to *practice them four times a day:* when you get up in the morning, around noon, in the late afternoon and before bedtime. These should be a part of your regular routine, just like brushing your teeth or washing your face. They are not something to do once in a while: you have to use them regularly to retain their benefits. You may have to be flexible at times with the schedule, as when you have a pressing chore that needs to be done at the times of day which you have allocated to practice, but try as much as possible to make relaxation a part of your routine.

Fifth, *never use these methods when you are driving.* The relaxation should be done in a very comfortable place, usually your bed or a chair, where you have no distractions. Let your family know that this is a part of your daily routine, and ask them not to disturb you at those times.

A last point that we would like to make has to do with the types of relaxation methods used. Although progressive muscle relaxation has been used very successfully to reduce anxiety, we do not recommend it for pain management because it involves systematically tensing and relaxing muscle groups which may be difficult on your body and may inadvertently hurt it in some cases.

We will only briefly describe the various techniques of meditation, autogenics, guided imagery, biofeedback and hypnosis. There is a great overlap between them, but they all help get you to deep relaxation states. It is not so important which one of these procedures you use or even what you call it as much as that you like this method and that it works for you. If you don't like it, you won't use it: so it is important to find something you enjoy and that you find useful.

All of these methods have the same goal in mind which is to get at some deep states of relaxation to alleviate your pain. All have some common features including the need for a quiet environment and a comfortable position, together with a passive "let it happen" attitude. All essentially involve focusing your attention away from external, distracting thoughts to inner relaxation.

Meditation is the practice of uncritically attempting to focus your attention on one thing at a time. It doesn't really matter what it is you try to focus on. A simple meditation involves breathing in and out and counting each breath as it occurs. Some people find this difficult to do when they try to keep count and may prefer to repeat the same word, such as "one" after each breath. *Benson's Relaxation Response* is essentially a meditation where a person relaxes his/her muscles and breathes in and out for ten to twenty minutes, saying the word "one" after each breath. What is most interesting about this relaxation method is that not only do people report feeling calmer afterwards but that *it has a direct effect on their body physiology,* essentially producing bodily changes such as decreased blood pressure that are the opposite of the physiological changes that occur when the body is under stress.

Autogenic Training, like meditation, also reverses the "fight or flight" or alarm state that occurs when the body experiences physical or emotional stress. It uses a series of standard visualization exercises directly oriented to body physiology. In a relaxed, comfortable state, persons concentrate on their bodies mentally or visually as they repeat statements that promote feelings of well-being in their body, such as "My right arm is heavy", "My arms and legs are warm", or "My heartbeat is calm and regular". After people have learned the six standard body exercises, they may go on to do a series of meditative exercises where they visualize colors, objects, concepts such as happiness or other people and can ask questions of their unconscious, inner self. Autogenic training is widely practiced in Europe and has been extensively researched. It has been used to treat a large number of diseases, including low back pain and headaches. The research on autogenic training suggests that it has very significant healing physiological changes, and that particular exercises may affect a specific organ or bodily process. Autogenic training has a lot in common with other visualization techniques including guided imagery and hypnosis.

Probably nowhere has the use of **guided imagery** been more dramatic than in the work with cancer patients. Dr. Carl Simonton, a radiologist who worked with cancer, and his then wife Stephanie Matthews-Simonton, have used visualization in the treatment of cancer with some success. They describe this in their book *Getting Well Again* (1978). First they had their patients relax, then they asked them to visualize their cancer, their immune system and their treatment. They encouraged their patients to use images that made the white blood cells and the treatment strong, conquering the weak cancer cells. For example, patients could visualize a strong army of white blood cells killing the cancer cells with the aid of the strong energy from their radiation treatment blasting away at the tumors. Patients were taught about how their immune system worked and how tumors healed so they could envision more accurately how their body worked and make their images more vivid and effective. They also confronted some of their negative beliefs about their cancer and replaced those with more positive ones.

The Simontons achieved very dramatic results with people using these methods. Of the patients who showed full cooperation, followed instructions implicitly and were enthusiastic about getting better, *nine out of nine* showed not only marked relief of symptoms but a dramatic improvement in their condition. Some tumors shrank markedly, some disappeared altogether, and some patients outlived their prognosis by many years. How do we explain these dramatic results? The Simontons concluded that a person's visualizations play a significant role in the cause and treatment of a disease.

The Simontons and others have used visualizations specifically designed for managing pain. These include imagining the body's healing resources, communicating with the pain and visualizing the pain. They encourage people to get inside the body to understand the difficulty and to then correct it. For example, they can see muscles relaxing like tight rubber bands going limp. Take some time to write down how you visualize your pain and your body's healing resources. You can draw it if you wish. Explore how you might incorporate that image into your relaxation.

_____

_____

_____

_____

_____

_____

_____

_____

A Picture of My Pain

The Simontons also ask their patients to communicate with their pain in this relaxed state and ask it what it wants from them. For example, your pain could be saying you are pushing yourself too hard or that you are not getting enough pleasure. When Bill talked to his pain, it told him: "Don't be John Wayne today". Ellen's pain told her: "Don't blame yourself or everything that goes wrong". Marge's pain told her: "Try to get more laughter in your life". Take a few minutes to close your eyes and picture what your pain looks like. Try to make it look like a creature and see if you can visualize it. Ask it what it is telling you and what you do to get rid of it. Write down your response after you open your eyes.

_____

_____

_____

_____

_____

_____

You can also visualize your pain and try to make the image go away. For example, if the pain is a large ball, you can shrink it to the size of a pea. Or if it is a bright red color, see if you can change it to a light pink. Or see if you can make it disappear as you move it away from your body, just as Jerry made the pain bubbles disappear from his consciousness as he was sitting in the dentist's chair.

Hypnosis is another powerful tool to use imagery to manage your pain. Although many people think of hypnosis as something mysterious, it is actually something we all do every day. Have you ever watched a movie and been so engrossed in it that you forgot your surroundings? Have you ever been so wrapped up in a novel that you were not aware of anything else? Have you ever driven from work to home while your mind was somewhere else? You got home somehow and made all the right turns and stopped at all the signals but your attention was elsewhere. If you have had any of these experiences, then you have been in a hypnotic state: your body was in one place and your mind was in another. Hypnosis is *focused attention:* attending fully to something to the exclusion of everything else.

There are many misconceptions about hypnosis, the first one being that someone does things to you and puts you under his or her spell. This is unfortunately reinforced by television and the movies. In truth, all hypnosis is self-hypnosis. Nobody can hypnotize you but they can teach you hypnosis to use in your own behalf. Hypnosis is a legitimate tool of the American Medical Association, the American Psychiatric and Psychological Associations, and the American Dental Association, all of whom use it in their practice. Medical hypnosis is different from stage hypnosis and is used in a wide variety of conditions, particularly pain.

Hypnosis is learned, and most people can learn it if they can concentrate and focus their attention. One of the leading authorities on hypnosis reported that when he used to work in a clinic that happened to be located at the bottom of a ski slope, everyone whom he treated for fractures and sprains learned to use hypnosis when it was the primary form of anesthesia! We have probably all witnessed hypnosis on pain with children.

How many of us can remember hearing, "Let Mommy kiss this booboo and make it better"?

In a state of deep hypnosis, people can use the power of suggestion to produce changes in their bodies. One very effective suggestion is to make the pain area numb. For example, you can imagine your hands getting numb and spread that sensation to other parts of your body. Or you can transfer the pain from one part of your body and have it all concentrate in one little area, like your finger. In hypnotherapy, many people have learned to imagine a light switch which they can use to turn off their pain. Children in particular have little difficulty turning off their pain switch. Distraction is another hypnotic technique, where a person can focus on a pleasant scene while surgery is taking place. So is picturing healing inside the body, as the Simontons and others have done. Hypnotherapy can be an excellent pain reliever, and there are many people who have undergone surgery with no other form of anesthesia. If you decide to learn self-hypnosis to lower your pain, be certain to go to a trained professional who has been certified by the American Society of Clinical Hypnosis and not just someone whose advertises on television and the newspaper.

Biofeedback is a term coined by persons using this method, which means providing the person with immediate information or *feedback* on the *biological* functions of his body. Through the aid of a biofeedback machine, a person can "see" or "hear" his body and learn to control, for example, his muscle tension. A tone goes up when muscles are tense and goes down when they are relaxed. People can thus learn to decrease the tension in their bodies. Biofeedback has been used for headaches and back pain, among other conditions. It can be combined with any of the other relaxation methods we have already talked about to give you control over your internal states and to lower your pain.

Developing Pain-Resistant Attitudes

Besides using our mind power to lower the pain, we can also learn to develop attitudes that can reduce it. We have already seen how negative emotions can open the pain gate and devastate our nervous system. There is a great deal of research which shows that stress can wear down the body's immune system, and that many people can and do develop illnesses following stressful periods. However, not everybody gets sick when they are under pressure. What distinguishes people who don't succumb to illness in spite of unusually stressful lives? Psychologist Suzanne Kobasa (1979, 1984), examined a group of executives who had experienced a highly stressful year but had not become ill and compared them to a similar group of men who did get sick. She found out that there were three characteristics that distinguished illness-resistant people from others. Hardiness or stress-resistance involves the three C's of *commitment, control, and challenge.*

Commitment means being connected rather than alienated. These men were all devoted to their jobs, their families and to other important values. They also had a sense of *control* and personal mastery over their lives. They did not see themselves as victims but believed that they could shape their fate. The third C- *challenge*—is seeing life changes not as threats but as chances to test themselves. Some of our presidents have been examples of hardy people. Although they have a great deal of stress in their lives, they withstand the long hours and the hard decisions they make because they have a commitment and sense of purpose. Their life has a meaning beyond the daily grind. They also have a feeling of control and believe they can make effective changes. They view the problems as a challenge rather than as a threat, frequently looking for new and creative solutions to domestic and foreign dilemmas.

A sense of *control* is probably one of the most important aspects of dealing with your pain. We have already talked about internal and external control in the first chapter and how it relates to health. Numerous studies have shown a clear relationship between the level of control and the amount of perceived pain. How people respond to pain—whether feeling in charge or like victims—makes a significant difference in how they cope with it. When people feel helpless, it affects the immune system in a terrible way. Rats in laboratory experiments who had some control over an electric shock which they could turn off by manipulating a lever respond very differently from rats who did not have control over their shocks. Those rats who had no lever learned to be helpless, and even in situations when they had a chance to escape, did not do so because of this learned helplessness. These "helpless" rats are much more prone to disease.

Human beings as well respond better to pain when they feel in control. For example, patients with terminal cancer use less medication when they have some control over the dosage. Some persons with chronic pain develop such a sense of helplessness, a "what's the use" attitude, that they don't even attempt to do things they could compared to others who see themselves as regular human beings with a problem—one that slows them down, to be sure—but does not have them licked.

Individuals who feel in control generally have a sense of optimism about their recovery whereas those who feel helpless are more pessimistic. A person can either say, "I'm a helpless victim of incurable pain, and I just have to learn to live with it" or "I will keep looking till I find something that will help". As Sherry said when her doctors told her there was nothing more they could do for her: "Just because they went to college doesn't mean they know everything. They have been wrong with me before and I don't have to accept this as a death sentence." Sherry also stated: "Maybe I can't control the pain as much as I want but I can control how I respond to it. I'm not just going to lay down and die. I won't allow it to ruin my life." Optimism, hope and control go hand in hand, and people can learn to change their pessimistic beliefs into ones that give them more of a sense of mastery in their lives.

"Isn't that being like Pollyanna?" some people ask. "You can't deny the pain—life stinks." It may be true that pain is here to stay but you do have a choice in how to respond to it. Pain and misery do not have to go hand in hand.

Developing a *commitment* to ourselves, our family and the larger community is very important to our well-being. An attitude that we are useful and have some meaning and purpose in life is essential. Lenny and Sherry, in spite of the debilitating effects of pain on their lives, still felt that they had responsibilities as parents and spouses. Focusing on a purpose or meaning that transcends the physical level—feeling that one is worthwhile and can contribute—these are very important attitudes to develop. We will explore this topic in greater depth in a later chapter.

The third attitude that can help in lowering your pain is that of seeing the *challenge* in the situation. Bill described this very well: "When it gets worse, it starts to make me more creative, and that's a challenge. The worse I get physically, the more I have to think about how to do this. Being creative is what will keep me afloat—to get me back on track." Bill has reframed his pain in a way that not only makes it bearable but also makes it a challenge to cope with.

Take a few minutes to take the Hardiness Test (Kobasa, 1984) to see how hardy you are:

HOW HARDY ARE YOU?

Below are 12 items similar to those that appear in the hardiness questionnaire. Evaluating someone's hardiness requires more than this quick test. But this simple exercise should give you some idea of how hardy you are.

Write down how much you agree or disagree with the following statements, using this scale:

0 = strongly disagree   2 = mildly agree
1 = mildly disagree   3 = strongly agree

____A. Trying my best at work makes a difference.

____B. Trusting to fate is sometimes all I can do in a relationship.

____C. I often wake up eager to start on the day's projects.

____D. Thinking of myself as a free person leads to great frustration and difficulty.

____E. I would be willing to sacrifice financial security in my work if something challenging came along.

____F. It bothers me when I have to deviate from the routine or schedule I've set for myself.

____G. An average citizen can have an impact on politics.

____H. Without the right breaks, it is hard to be successful in my field.

____I. I know why I am doing what I'm doing at work.

____J. Getting close to people puts me at risk of being obligated to them.

____K. Encountering new situations is an important priority in my life.

____L. I really don't mind when I have nothing to do.

To Score Yourself: These questions measure control, commitment and challenge. For half the questions, a high score (like 3, "strongly agree") indicates hardiness; for the other half, a low score (disagreement) does.

To get your scores on **control, commitment** and **challenge,** first write in the number of your answers above the letter of each question on the score sheet. Then add and subtract as shown. (To get your score on "control," for example, add your answers to questions A and G; add your answers to B and H; and then subtract the second number from the first.)

Add your scores on commitment, control and challenge together to get a **Total Hardiness Score.**

A total score of 10-18 shows a hardy personality. 0-9 = moderate hardiness. Below 0 = low hardiness.

____+____= ____
A   G

____+____= - ____
B   H

____ **Control Score**

____+____= ____
C   I

____+____= - ____
D   J

____ **Commitment Score**

____+____= ____
E   K

____+____= - ____
F   L

____   **Challenge Score**

_____ + _____ + _____ = _____

Control   **Commitment**   **Challenge**   **Total Hardiness Score**

How does a person with chronic pain develop hardiness? Look at your responses to the test, and evaluate how you can add more control, commitment and challenge to your life. Let us look at each of these in turn.

Control: Do I determine my own limits or do I let others do that for me? Do I tell people what my needs are? Do I feel like a victim or do I believe that I have a choice in how I am responding to my situation? Am I actively participating in my own health or am I leaving it up to others? What do I need to do to gain more control over my life?

_____

_____

_____

_____

_____

_____

_____

_____

_____

_____

_____

Commitment: Do I have a commitment to my health? Do I maintain healthy habits? Do I get involved in causes I believe in? Do I approach life with a sense of purpose? Do I surround myself with positive people? Do I engage in activities that make me feel useful? What can I do to add more meaning to my life right now? We will talk about this in more depth in a later chapter, but right now we would like you to think of more ways to commit yourself to people and things you believe in.

_____

_____

_____

_____

_____

_____

_____

_____

Challenge: How do I handle change? How can I learn to look for growth in change? How can I turn this problem into a challenge rather than an obstacle? Can I learn to make lemonade if life has handed me a lemon?

_____

_____

_____

_____

_____

_____

_____

_____

Changing the Way You Think About Pain

Before we talk about changing some of your attitudes about pain, we would like you to take some time to explore your beliefs about pain and how they could be affecting you today. In the space below, answer the following questions:

What are my beliefs about pain?

_____

_____

_____

_____

_____

_____

_____

_____

How did my family deal with pain?

_____

_____

_____

_____

What is my religious background, and how do I view pain and suffering with that context?

_____

_____

_____

_____

Do I perceive pain as suffering, as a punishment, as a friend?

_____

_____

_____

_____

_____

Your answers can help illuminate your thinking for you and help you make some changes.

It is not so much the pain but also the *meaning* we give to it that can affect us. Mary felt shame whenever she became aware of the burning in her groin, reminding her of her affair last summer which brought on the venereal disease. Karen sometimes delighted in the pains she felt in her belly when her baby kicked—each movement reminded her that her baby was alive and well.

How we *interpret* our pain can increase its discomfort or reduce it. "I can't always control my pain but I can control my attitude about it," Sherry told us. "It's not always easy. I know many times that pain is unavoidable but I don't have to make myself miserable". Bill too shared these sentiments: "I try to stay away from the negative stuff and go to the positive. It doesn't get rid of my pain but my attitude is all right."

Sherry and Bill are trying as much as possible to separate the pain from their happiness. Many people see pain as the enemy, something that has destroyed their lives and to be gotten rid of at all costs. Dr. Paul Brand who worked for years with lepers in India has written eloquently about the positive effects of pain. Without the sensations of pain to guide them, these lepers lost fingers because they had no warning that something was wrong. Dr. Brand suggests "befriending pain": to take what is seen as an enemy and making it a friend. He recommends having an attitude of gratitude towards pain. As he tells his patients: "Think of pain as a speech your body is delivering about a subject of vital importance to you." He further adds that the body is using the language of pain because that is the most effective way to get their attention. Gratitude may seem like the last attitude that you want to develop about your pain, but as Dr. Brand reminds us, even in bodily processes normally regarded as enemies, we can find a reason to be grateful. Nearly every bodily activity that we view with irritation is an emblem of the body's self-protection.

Whether you choose to befriend pain or not, you do not have to allow it to get the best of you. The following is a table of some of the statements that you may be telling yourself. On the left are ones which make the pain worse. On the right are some more appropriate thoughts that will help you cope better.

CHANGING THE WAY YOU THINK ABOUT PAIN

Review these statements and check the ones you use.

Negative Thoughts	Positive Thoughts
☐ "Why me? It's not fair!"	☐ "Life isn't always fair but I can learn to manage this."
☐ "I'm a helpless victim of pain and I just have to live with it."	☐ "I'll keep looking till I find something that helps."
☐ "I hate this—it stinks."	☐ "I'm not going to add to my pain by being miserable as well."
☐ "This has ruined my life."	☐ "I can't always control my pain but I can control my attitude about it."
☐ "I can't do anything anymore."	☐ "I need to concentrate on the things I *can* do."
☐ "What's the use?"	☐ "If I act like a victim, I will feel worse."
☐ "It gets worse every day."	☐ "I just have to find more creative ways to manage it."
☐ "My pain has taken over my life."	☐ "I'm a person with a problem. My pain does slow me down but it doesn't have to take over my life."

Negative Thoughts	**Positive Thoughts**
	☐ "I can learn ways to manage my pain."
	☐ "How can I make the best out of this situation?"
	☐ "It's not so much my limitations but the way I think about them."
☐ "I'm not a man/woman or father/mother anymore."	☐ "Being a spouse or parent involves caring, not just caretaking."
☐ "I'm no good to anyone any more."	☐ "I'm a human *being,* not a human 'doing'."
☐ "It hurts so much!"	☐ "Let me listen to what my body is trying to tell me."
	☐ "One step at a time."
	☐ "Relax and take a deep breath."
	☐ "Don't try to get rid of the pain entirely—just keep it under control."
	☐ "My pain is my ally, telling me what I need to do."

What other statements do you tell yourself that make your pain worse? Write those down.

_____

_____

_____

_____

_____

_____

_____

_____

_____

_____

_____

How can you replace these statements with better coping statements?

_____

_____

_____

_____

_____

_____

_____

_____

_____

_____

_____

_____

Stress
Negative Imagery
Negative Attitudes
Negative Thoughts

PAIN

Relaxation
Positive Imagery
Positive Attitudes
Positive Thoughts

PAIN

Changing the Way You Think About Yourself

Not only do we need to change the way we think about pain, we need to change the way we think about ourselves as persons with pain. As we have seen throughout this book, pain affects all aspects of our lives and hits at the very core of our being. Who am I now if I am no longer a provider, coach, athlete? As Lenny succinctly described it: "I'm a changed man." The pain crisis affects how we define ourselves *(self-concept)* and how we evaluate ourselves *(self-esteem)*.

Our *self-concept* develops from our encounters, and we have different ways to describe ourselves depending on the roles we play. In response to the question, "Who am I?" one can respond: "Truckdriver, father, husband, native Arizonan, Catholic, good basketball player, mediocre swimmer, outgoing, handsome, funny, responsible." Our self-definitions come from the *roles* we play and also from characteristics that make us distinct from others. Our *self-esteem* or how much we value ourselves frequently comes from the way we describe ourselves.

Since so much of our self-worth derives from the roles we play, when we can no longer perform certain functions, we start to ask ourselves "Who am I?" and frequently translate that to "What good am I?" Both self-concept and self-esteem are affected when there is a change in what we can do. We have already talked about how much of our self-worth is derived from our *roles*, our *doing* instead of our *being*. However, who we are is more than the roles we play and more than the physical aspects of ourselves. When we talk about the self and attempt to answer the question of "Who am I?", we need to look at the *essence* of who we are, the qualities that surpass the physical being. Before we look further at this, take a few minutes to answer the following simple question:

Who am I?

_____

_____

_____

_____

_____

_____

_____

_____

_____

_____

_____

_____

_____

_____

   How does your description reflect your self-concept and how you feel about yourself?

_____

_____

_____

_____

_____

_____

_____

_____

_____

_____

_____

_____

_____

How many of your descriptions are qualities that are uniquely you, that go beyond the physical realm? Write those down.

_____

_____

_____

_____

_____

_____

_____

_____

_____

It is very important to keep in mind that you are more than all of the different roles you play, that *although everything else in your life has changed, your basic self, is intact. Pain has not made you a changed person. You are the same person—with pain.* Many persons with chronic pain have let pain define who they are, and it is frequently one of their first self-descriptions. Look back to your response to the question "Who am I?" If you have put your illness or injury at the beginning of the list (e.g. "I'm an arthritic," "I'm disabled," etc.), you have probably allowed pain to change your feelings about yourself.

When Marion developed genital warts, she could not attend to anything else except the burning sensations in her body. She tried to focus on other aspects of her life but the discomfort of the symptoms was primary in her mind. Her self-esteem was shattered because her venereal disease also reminded her of her marital infidelity and her reckless behavior. She felt that she was worthless and deserved to be punished for what she did. She was also very angry at the pain. Marion's doctor noticed the way in which she had let her symptoms permeate her life. He took her aside and reminded her that she was a beautiful woman, a capable professional, as well as intelligent, creative and generous. "Marion", he said to her, *"you are acting like you are one big wart."*

If, like Marion, you are feeling as though you are "one big wart", then it is important to remind yourself that you are more than your symptoms. Take a few minutes to write down all of your positive qualities.

_____

_____

_____

_____

_____

_____

_____

_____

_____

_____

Remember, underneath all of the physical barriers, you are still the same person you have always been. As Cheri Register writes: "I think of myself as a very healthy person—with a problem" (p.27). Don't let pain define who you are or how you feel about yourself!

Summary

You can use your mind as an ally to help you lower your pain and its negative effect on your life. First, there are a number of very effective relaxation and imagery techniques which you can employ, but these have to be learned thoroughly and to be practiced four times a day to be of benefit to you. Secondly, you can develop the attitudes of control, commitment and challenge which can make you more pain resistant. Thirdly, you can change the way you think about pain and its effect on your self-image and decrease its negative impact on your life. Even if you cannot avoid your pain at times, you can avoid feeling miserable.

Chapter 8

Interpersonal Aspects of Pain & Pain Management

"No man is an island."

In the preceding chapters, we had talked about how pain affects the person who has it. In this chapter we will talk about how it affects relationships with others: family, friends and loved ones.

Marriage: In Sickness & In Health

The marriage vow "In sickness and in health" also translates into "for poorer" and "for worse" in the case of many partners of persons with chronic pain. It is not only the pain sufferers who feel cheated out of life, as Lenny did, but their spouses as well. Both partners feel cheated and frustrated. Many persons with chronic pain start to think that they did not live up to their part of the marriage bargain. They experience shame at being deficient partners and that they are bringing less to the marital relationship than their mates. They feel like a burden to their families, and many frequently wonder why their spouses stay with them. They become guilty about their plight and get withdrawn and irritable. Spouses often are helpless to deal with the situation. They find it difficult to see their partners hurting as well and don't know how to intervene. They also become angry and resentful for getting less than they bargained for and for having to take on an extra load. Like their partners, they experience losses too: of a lifestyle, of many pleasurable experiences together—and of the man or woman they married. They feel guilty about their feelings and may withdraw from the partner and the situation.

The experience is sometimes different for men and women. Many men, like Lenny, may feel humiliated at not being the provider but it is okay to have the wife as caretaker. As he said,

"We're old-fashioned: she does the laundry; I do the cars". Women feel shame at not being able to be caretakers, which is what they frequently see as their role. They believe they should be taking care of the loved ones, not the other way around!

These feelings of resentment, anger, helplessness and frustration are not always talked about openly. In addition, the loss of income and medical and legal expenses can cause a further rift in the marital relationship. The divorce rate for pain patients is very high, between 60 and 80 percent, according to Norman Shealy, "indicating that the worse of 'for better or for worse' does not often include chronic pain" (p.5).

Ellen's family found it very difficult to be around her. As she told us, "My husband couldn't stand to see me sick. We used to do a lot of things together and also as a family. Now they all go out without me. They used to ask me to join them at first but they don't even do that anymore. They just make plans without me and go on with their lives. My children are tired of hearing me say, 'Mommy can't'."

Lenny's family, on the other hand, did not ignore him and go off on their own merry way. When he stopped riding his bike, they stopped going riding as well. If he couldn't do something, they stopped doing it as well—and became isolated with him in the process.

Ellen and Lenny's families responded the way many families do. The following diagram "Family Response to Pain" illustrates what often happens in families of persons with chronic pain. The person in pain may talk about his or her pain which may make family members uncomfortable and powerless to help him or her. They get tired of hearing about the pain and engage in one of two patterns: they either all withdraw together or they go about their lives, abandoning the person with pain. In one case, they will say, "Since you can't ride a bike, go to the movies, picnic or whatever, we'll stay home with you". In the other case, they will not let him or her "spoil their fun" and go on with their lives while he or she feels more isolated and sinks further and further into depression. In some situations, the spouse may leave altogether.

Whether the family abandons the chronic pain person or

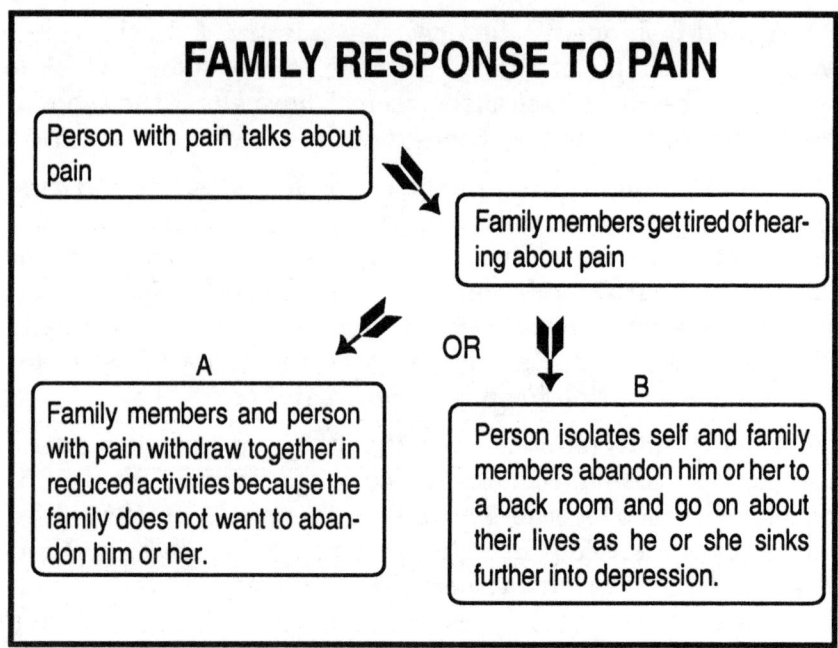

FAMILY RESPONSE TO PAIN

Person with pain talks about pain

Family members get tired of hearing about pain

A OR **B**

Family members and person with pain withdraw together in reduced activities because the family does not want to abandon him or her.

Person isolates self and family members abandon him or her to a back room and go on about their lives as he or she sinks further into depression.

withdraws with him or her, neither pattern is really satisfactory, and in both cases the person feels more isolated and alone. If you or your family is engaged in one of these patterns or another pattern that is not working for you, it is important to talk about that candidly. When people communicate their feelings openly, they can frequently negotiate and resolve these problems.

In the space below write down:

What is my family's response to my pain?

_____

_____

_____

_____

_____

_____

_____

How can I improve communication between me and my spouse?

_____

_____

_____

_____

_____

_____

_____

_____

How can I improve my communication with my children?

_____

_____

_____

_____

_____

_____

_____

If you are a parent of younger children, you may be worried about how your children view you. Many parents feel guilty that they can't do things with or for their children. Lenny could not play basketball with his son; Sherry could not go to the movies with her children or take care of them the way she would have liked. We have to remember that *caring* for our children is not the same as *caretaking*. Caring has two components: loving and taking care of, being and doing. Pain does not take away your ability to love. There are other ways to show love to your children besides taking them fishing or cooking their favorite meals. The same of course goes for your spouse!

In the space below, write down all of the ways in which you can show love and caring to your family that do not involve physical "doing":

_____

_____

_____

_____

_____

_____

_____

_____

_____

_____

_____

_____

Pain and Sex: The Agony & the Ecstasy

One of the areas that is affected in a marital relationship when there is chronic pain is that of intimacy, sexual and otherwise. Frequently, the person with pain may not know the cause of the pain and fears that sexual activity may hurt the body and result in more pain. In addition, depression causes further loss of sexual desires. When people are feeling depressed, they do not enjoy the things that used to give them pleasure.

There is another reason why sex often goes out the window when there is chronic pain, and that is that sometimes people don't feel like they are "a man" or "a woman" any longer. Lenny for example did not view himself as "a real man" if he could no longer support his wife and do the activities which defined his sexual role. Similarly, a woman who is not able to perform her role as wife or mother in the traditional sense may feel that she is "not a complete woman." Persons with pain frequently see themselves as being "less than"—as inadequate.

Another reason why sexuality is affected when there is chronic pain is the self-hate and particularly hate for the body when it is not working properly. Sometimes the weight gain from the inactivity causes the person with pain to loathe the body even more and to feel shame about it. To love oneself and one's body is very important for healthy sexuality. Unfortunately, in chronic pain that is not often the case.

Melanie and John had a very active and very satisfactory sex life before she started experiencing pain. However, they have almost stopped having sexual relations since her accident. Melanie feels very guilty about it, especially when her husband brings up how much he misses her. "He's usually pretty good but the other night he told me, 'You know, it's been nearly two months since we had any sex.' I just felt so bad and so guilty."

"I don't feel like a woman anymore", she continued. "I also miss having sex with him but it hurts so much afterwards, that I'm afraid to even start anything so I don't touch him or rub against him or stroke him or do anything that might get him excited because I know what will happen afterwards. He's really been pretty good too—he waits for me to make a move. He doesn't touch me or try to arouse me. He's real considerate but I know it's hard for him. We just don't show as much affection as we used to and I miss it."

Melanie and John depict what frequently happens sexually when there is chronic pain. The person with chronic pain is afraid that having sex is going to hurt. It's hard to think of sex when you fear that you may hurt afterwards for the next few days. The spouse as well is afraid to ask for sex knowing it may hurt his or her partner—so both stop asking. However, it doesn't just end there. Both "don't want to start anything they can't finish" so the hugging and cuddling which are a very important component of affection cease. Sometimes all physical contact halts because it might lead to sex and sex could result in pain. At times, even verbal affection ceases because that could culminate in physical affection and physical affection could end up in sex which can become painful. "I'm afraid to be emotionally close because that could lead to a series of steps which could lead to sex: so I avoid it altogether," a spouse told us. Unfortunately, what may happen in even very loving relationships is the complete cessation of verbal and physical intimacy. The following table depicts this cycle.

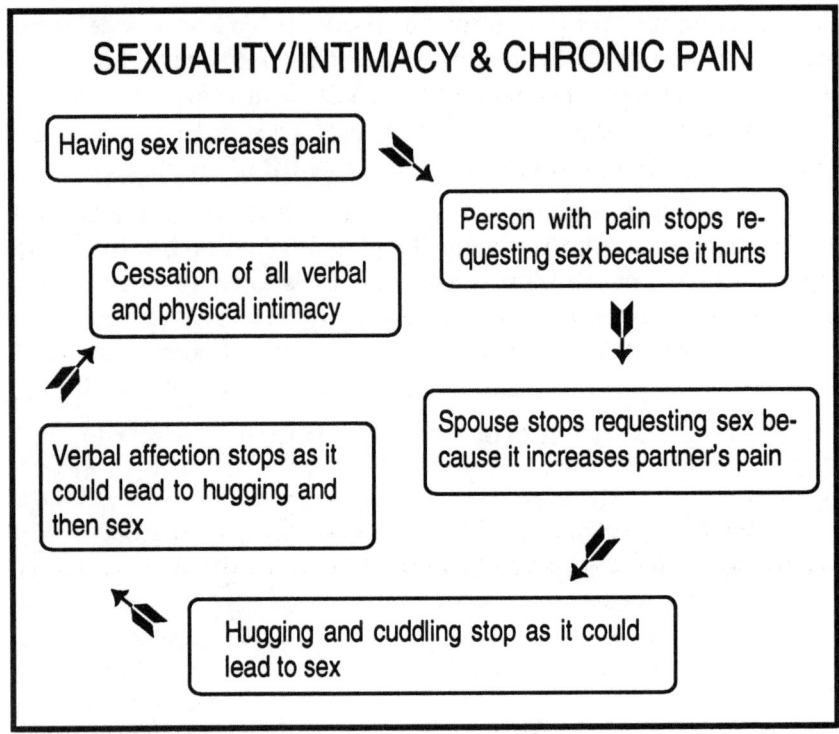

SEXUALITY/INTIMACY & CHRONIC PAIN

- Having sex increases pain
- Person with pain stops requesting sex because it hurts
- Cessation of all verbal and physical intimacy
- Spouse stops requesting sex because it increases partner's pain
- Verbal affection stops as it could lead to hugging and then sex
- Hugging and cuddling stop as it could lead to sex

This cycle does not need to happen. Having sex does not have to lead to pain, and in sexual relations, as with every other physical activity, principles of proper positioning are important. Many persons do not educate themselves about what they can comfortably do and therefore deprive themselves of further pleasure and intimacy. The first thing to do whether you are a person with pain or a spouse is to educate yourself about the pain and eliminate some of your fears about it. Proper communication between you and your partner is essential, and you may need to talk to a counselor about this together. The improvement of general communications between you has to be the most important goal, together with relieving your anxiety about having sex.

Many people have certain misconceptions about sex that need to be clarified, the most important one being that sex and sexual intercourse are one and the same. Sexuality and intimacy are more than the mechanics of pelvic thrusting. Sex does not only relate to the genitals or traditional intercourse but has to do with loving, hugging and touching that can involve other bodily organs and positions. The standard missionary position is not the only way to have sex, and manual and oral pleasuring can be performed if intercourse puts a strain on muscles. There are ways to be loving without hurting.

Physical and emotional intimacy are vital to your emotional well-being and to your marriage, and you need to discuss together how you can continue to make that source of pleasure primary in your relationship. If sex is important to you and your partner, you will need to manage it like you do other areas of your life. As Bill told us, "When I feel good, I get the drive. I have to plan for it, just like I do for everything else, like going to the music festival in Flagstaff or anything else I want to do . I have to rest, pace myself and do what I love even if I don't do it as much as I did before. I do what I can within my limitations. My mental attitude is what keeps me on track. It's the fear that may get me down." Bill was voicing a very real truth—it is not so much the physical aspects of sexuality that may bring on pain—it is the *fear and anxiety* about its consequences. That is the first step in the cycle. Before we give you some sexual tips, take some time to write down in the space below some of your concerns and fears about sex. You may wish to involve your partner in this.

_____

_____

_____

_____

_____

_____

_____

_____

_____

_____

_____

_____

_____

_____

The following table provides some suggestions to resume and/or enhance your sexual relations:

SUGGESTIONS FOR COMFORTABLE SEX

1. Eat lightly and limit alcohol consumption
2. Do not mix pain medication and alcohol.
3. Pace yourself—slow down in life and slow down in sex.
4. Exercise regularly for good muscle tone including pelvis tilt.
5. Practice relaxation exercises four times a day to maintain muscles in a relaxed state.
6. Use proper body mechanics when sitting, kneeling, lifting and getting up to keep strain at a minimum.
7. Take medication on a time contingent basis.
8. Do *not* use transcutaneous neural stimulators (TENS) during sex to prevent sudden electrical jolts if wires come loose.
9. Maintain proper nutrition for good body image and less strain to the muscles and joints.
10. Take a warm bath to loosen muscles.
11. Use body positions during sex that put minimal strain on your body.

In sexual relations, as with every other physical activity, the principles of sensible care and mechanics hold true. In your particular situation, try to determine which positions are most comfortable for you and exert the least strain on your body. However, even if at times no position seems comfortable, *do not give up the hugging, cuddling and physical intimacy.* Physical and emotional nourishment are the life blood of relationships. Just as a plant cannot survive without water, we can not survive without affection.

Sexual relations, using sensible positions, can be good for your back. Dr. Leon Root (1985) describes an incident in which one of his fellow interns who had twisted his back and was in considerable pain, dragged himself to a party where he lay down in a quiet corner and was feeling in pain and incapacitated. The next morning, the young man came to work looking comfortable, his back straight and walking without any difficulty. When he was asked how he accounted for this dramatic turnabout in his condition, he replied "Worked it out last night". As Dr. Root states: "The gentle push-pull thrusts of the pelvis during sexual intercourse not only contribute to sexual pleasure and fulfillment, they can also be good therapy for an ailing back if done properly. Keep that in mind next time you are reluctant about having sex because of your fear of back pain" (p.211).

There are other instances where sexual pleasure can actually decrease pain. For example, many woman report that having an orgasm reduces menstrual cramps. In addition, orgasms can be an antidote for migraine headaches. Many people have reported that their migraines went away following an orgasm where blood accumulates in the pelvic area instead of the head. Keep that in mind the next time you don't have sex because you have a headache—sex may help you get rid of the headache!

People Who Need People . . .

We all need people in our lives, particularly when we are hurting. Tragically, many persons with chronic pain withdraw from others and feel more and more isolated. Lenny, if you recall, said that you could put him into a room with many others, and he would not say a word. Whether persons in pain are shut off from family in a back room by themselves or whether the rest of the family serves as a protective cocoon as they *all* shut themselves off, the person's world becomes more and more limited. As Mary Sarton (1980) states, "In the country of pain, we are each alone."

People with chronic pain shut themselves off from other people for many reasons. First of all, pain is an energy drain. It takes tremendous effort just to keep going and keep oneself healthy. Many people with chronic pain are fatigued and just do not have the physical and emotional energy to keep a friendship going. As one woman said, "Sometimes I just can't be in shape to give anything to anyone or to give what it takes to be a friend."

Other reasons for the isolation are that some people don't want their friends to see them in their weak moments and to feel sorry for them. They are afraid that they will be seen as "babies". They still would like others to view them as strong and independent, and not as helpless and weak. There is also a reluctance to bother others and burden them with their problems. Which one of their friends will they allow to look at them in this raw shape, without the protective social layers? Letting people view your hurt involves a strong level of intimacy, and many persons find it humiliating to be seen at their worst.

Some people perceive emotional involvement with people as making them more vulnerable to hurt. As Bill said: "I don't want to bother anybody and I don't want anybody to bother me because anything—just emotions—it affects me—even now—you can't see it but underneath my skin, stuff is starting to form."

Dora disagrees with Bill: "As long as I have breath, I feel I have to have emotional involvement. I have to reach out to people. Life is about people and people is about problems and people is about knowing and loving and caring."

For Bill, people means more pain. For Dora, we cannot live without other people—problems and all. Although people like Bill insulate themselves from others for their protection, we all need other people, and the research supports this. *Loneliness kills*—literally—and loneliness can make us ill. There are dozens of studies that show the effects of loneliness on health. For example, married men tend to be healthier and live longer than their divorced and widowed counterparts. When a man loses his wife, his risk of dying earlier increases tremendously, although a woman who loses her husband doesn't increase her risk. Women usually have a network of friends that can still provide support. When a man's wife dies, he is not only losing his best friend—but often his only friend as well.

Studies have shown that social support is one of the most effective ingredients in getting well and lack of it in getting sick. Those who have strong social ties are more likely to be resistant to disease and to live longer. In a study of two groups of women with breast cancer, it was found that those women who were in a cancer support group as well lived much longer than those who didn't have a support group.

There are numerous studies which suggest that friendship is good for your health and can lower your pain. Even though it may be tempting to isolate yourself from others, remind yourself that friendship heals. It is good for your emotional health, and it is good for your physical health. If you are isolating yourself from others, you can start to call people. Just calling and saying hello is not going to involve much physical strain. Make some plans to get together with friends. It does not have to involve a strenuous activity. If meeting for a cup of coffee is all that you can manage right now, at least you will be drinking your coffee with others. Join a support group, one which encourages healthy expression of feelings rather than one that either forces you to "stuff" them by only accepting platitudes or one that lets you "marinate in your toxic anger".

One of the most helpful things you can do is some volunteer work. Helping others is one of the best ways to get outside yourself and feel useful. One volunteer described her experience as "being like Santa Claus 365 days out of the year." Many volunteers would agree with that statement. One of the best things you can do for your emotional and physical well-being is to "open the heart".

In the space below, write down some ways in which you can increase your involvement with others:

_____

_____

_____

_____

_____

_____

_____

_____

_____

_____

_____

_____

_____

Summary

Pain not only affects our relationship to ourselves but our relationship to others: our families and friends. In this chapter, we discuss ways of breaking the vicious cycle of isolation from others and achieving more intimacy. Friendship and love are necessary ingredients of healing.

Chapter 9

Finding Meaning in Life in Spite of the Pain

"Although the world is full of suffering, it is also full of overcoming it."

Helen Keller, *Optimism*

What do you do when pain has pulled the carpet out from under your life? In the first chapter, we described at length the problems that Lenny and others experience when they can no longer do the same job, engage in the same activities and be the same person they were before. We talked about the different stages in grieving for these losses, starting with the shock or denial and going through the roller coaster of emotions till there is an acceptance. How do we get to that point of acceptance and find meaning in life in spite of the pain? *Can* one do that?

In the preceding chapters, we have attempted to walk you through some of the stages of loss and provide you with practical tools to manage your pain and your life. By now, you may have learned to pace yourself and let go of intense destructive feelings that increase your pain. Where do you go from here? Can a person find meaning in life when everything around him has been changed and taken away?

Gary worked as the head of a printing press before his accident. Although he was a very devoted husband and father, he did not see his family very much because his work took up most of his time. The pressures of having to get a paper out to meet deadlines meant many evenings away from home. Gary would have proudly described himself as a workaholic, and his identity was strongly tied up with his career. After the accident, Gary could no longer work at his job and had to go on social security disability. Following a long and painstaking struggle, he learned to control his pain and to maintain a different type of life. Since he had always liked photography, he started spending more time on this hobby. He was also home a lot more, and even though he had missed out on his children's early years because of his work, he now could enjoy his grandchildren. He also had time to read, write and engage in some hobbies he didn't have time for before.

Living in the Present

Gary's new life was quiet and gratifying but it was difficult for him to enjoy it because *he kept comparing himself to what he used to be before the injury.* "I used to make a lot of money", he said. "I used to have a great job, I used to be able to do so much, and now look at me—I am living off disability, I can't work, I can't do half of what I used to do." Every time that Gary thought of how he used to be, he felt miserable. Unfortunately, Gary was being so upset by what he wasn't doing, he was missing out on what he was doing. Gary's focusing on the past was only taking away from his enjoying the present. He needed to see his new life as a different existence, a different type of life. As long as he was telling himself that's what life should be or ought to be, he was spoiling the here and now.

Gary realized that the reason he was miserable was that he was comparing himself now to how he was before the injury. He had to *change his reference point* and compare his present life now to what it was before he had treatment, when he was feeling helpless, isolated and in such pain that he couldn't do anything. He needed to make *that* his new reference point. Everything after that is better, and he may even be able to appreciate his new life. "I guess I've really come a long way, haven't I?" he said, when he viewed what his life was like immediately after the injury. "I'm no longer locked up in a room, I'm no longer in as much pain as I was before, I can do some things, and I can even do some things that are enjoyable."

Gary had to *learn to appreciate the new life* which was different from the old one but had to be enjoyed in its own right. At this point, for better or for worse, this is the new path. Nobody could of course take away from Gary what he had already accomplished, but he had to let go of the old life and focus on making the present as meaningful as possible. We need to ask ourselves, as Gary did, "What can I do to make this new life as good as it can be?" This is easier said than done, of course, and not everyone is able to do it, but as long as you can, you are ahead of the game.

Acceptance is not easy and is often frustrating. As one character in a recent film put it: "Why should I go to physical therapy? It's so boring! You do the same thing over and over again to learn to do something you could do before but did much better." Acceptance means knowing you can't go back to doing something you did before and better but focusing on the here and now. It means knowing your physical limits and then choosing a life that fits your needs within those boundaries. It is living as well as possible within those parameters. As one woman eloquently stated: "You can't banish the pain, but you don't need to make the most of it. Make the most of other things instead."

Acceptance is not a Pollyannaish denial of the illness nor a welcoming of the suffering, but as Cheri Register puts it: "What 'acceptance' really means then is taking responsibility for constructing a life in the spaces between those moments of dysfunction and adopting habits that will keep them to a minimum in intensity and frequently" (p.181). It is exercising what control you have realistically over how you live and coping as well as possible within those areas you cannot control.

Lisa, a woman with cancer who lost her home, her car, her mobility and independence, tried to make the most of her current situation instead of focusing on the past. She had many days of intense pain when she could not do much, and it was hard for her to keep her spirits up during those times. She was asked to write down how she found meaning in life in spite of the pain. This is what she wrote: "When I was asked to write about finding meaning in life, it occurred to me that God is more interested in how I live than how I die. I think I have been in the throes of 'poor me—ain't it awful' lately and I think it's time to turn this around: I decided that (1) I'll first call Tina and ask her to bring that form which I can mail to my congressman which would make a change in our environment, (2) I'll invite her over for a steak dinner, and we'll open the bottle of wine that Linda brought me, (3) I'll get a rubber band to put on my wrist and pull it when I have a negative thought, and (4) I'll plan visualization time every day."

Achieving Growth Through Pain

When Lisa focused on finding meaning in life, she recognized that in spite of her limitations, she could still make some contributions in this world by writing to her congressman, could still enjoy good food, wine and friends, and that focusing on the past only made her feel worse. Finding a meaning and a purpose in life is a daily choice. Acceptance has to do with *coping*, with trying to stay on top and find a purpose when life is difficult. As the saying goes, all boats sail smoothly in calm waters. It is in stormy weather that we have to learn to cope. How can we transform the pain crisis into a meaningful life?

In the first chapter, we asked you to look at the Good Grief cycle and to study the stages where you have been stuck, as well as the ways you have kept yourself stuck. Please go back to that chapter and review questions 1 and 2 again. What do I still need to do to deal with the loss?

_____

_____

_____

_____

_____

_____

_____

_____

_____

_____

Reread your responses to questions 3 and 4 which ask you for ways you have used to get out of stages where you are stuck and the strength you have to offer yourself and others because of your crisis. Take a few minutes to write down what additional strengths and coping strategies you have that have helped you deal with difficult situations in your life before.

_____

_____

_____

_____

_____

_____

_____

_____

_____

_____

In troublesome times, most of us have the ability to recover from the traumas and to turn the pain and energy of that experience into something worthwhile. However, change is seldom easy, and we try to hold on to the safety and security of what was before. When our lives, our identities and everything we know change around us, we are filled with terror, and yet in order to go on to the next stage , we have to let go of what was.

This terror of transitions is expressed very poignantly in this essay from which we have taken some excerpts:

> "Sometimes, I feel that my life is a series of trapeze swings. I'm either hanging on to a trapeze bar swinging along or, for a few moments in my life, I'm hurling across space in between bars. Most of the time, I spend my life hanging on for dear life to my trapeze-bar-of-the-moment...........In my heart-of-hearts I know that for me to grow, I must release my grip on this present, well-known bar to move on to the new one.....I know that I must totally release my grasp on my old bar, and for some moment in time, I must hurtle across space before I can grab onto the new bar. Each time I am filled with terror........And so for an eternity that can last a micro-second or a thousand lifetimes, I soar across the dark void of the 'past is gone, the future is not yet here'. It's called transition...... Whether or not my hunch is true, it remains that the transition zones in our lives are incredibly rich places. They should be honored, even savored. Yes, with all this pain and fear and

feelings of being out-of-control that can (but not necessarily) accompany transitions they are still the most alive, most growth filled, passionate, expansive moments of our lives."

(Author Unknown)

How can we use this transition zone in our best interests? How can we take the identity crisis that pain frequently brings on and transform that experience into a new meaningful life? In times of crisis, most of us have the innate capacity to recover from devastating problems and can readjust to life not only as well as but even better than before the trauma. It is said that when one door closes in life, another new door can open. Gary's new life, for example, enabled him to spend time with his wife, his children and grandchildren and to devote time to photography and new hobbies. Other people talk about having "time to smell the flowers". Take a few minutes to write down some ways in which you can transform your pain experience into something meaningful. Is there anything in your new life that you can appreciate?

_____

_____

_____

_____

_____

_____

_____

_____

Achieving a meaningful life is not just getting rid of the pain and suffering. It is also adding positive experiences to our lives. We need to strive to not just reduce the pain and negativity but to go towards wellness. Health is not only an absence of illness: it is filled with positive relationships, enjoyable activities, fun and making a contribution to life through work or volunteer work which makes life worthwhile, as you can see in the chart on health and wellness.

HEALTH AND WELLNESS

+5	Work/Volunteer Work
+4	Love, Positive Relationships, Adequate Rest
+3	Fun, New Hobbies and Activities
+2	Positive Attitude, Positive Thoughts, Love of Self, Love of Others
+1	
0	Pain Reduction
-1	Depression Reduction
-2	
-3	Pain and Suffering
-4	Depression, Anger, Resentfulness
-5	Isolation, Alone, Purposelessness

In the space below, write down at least 10 new hobbies that you would like to try that would give you pleasure:

1. _____

2. _____

3. _____

5. _____

6. _____

7. _____

8. _____

9. _____

10. _____

If You Can't Have Quantity, Then Have Quality

When we talk about health, we are not necessarily talking about being physically healthy but emotionally, mentally and spiritually sound as well. Being well and whole transcends physical limitations. It may be true that in your new life, you may be more physically limited than you were before, but that does not necessarily mean it has to be *worse*. If you can't have quantity, then focus on the *quality*. How can you make the most of what you have? It is sometimes only during crises that we stop and take a look at what is really important to us. Whether it's learning to appreciate the little things we took for granted

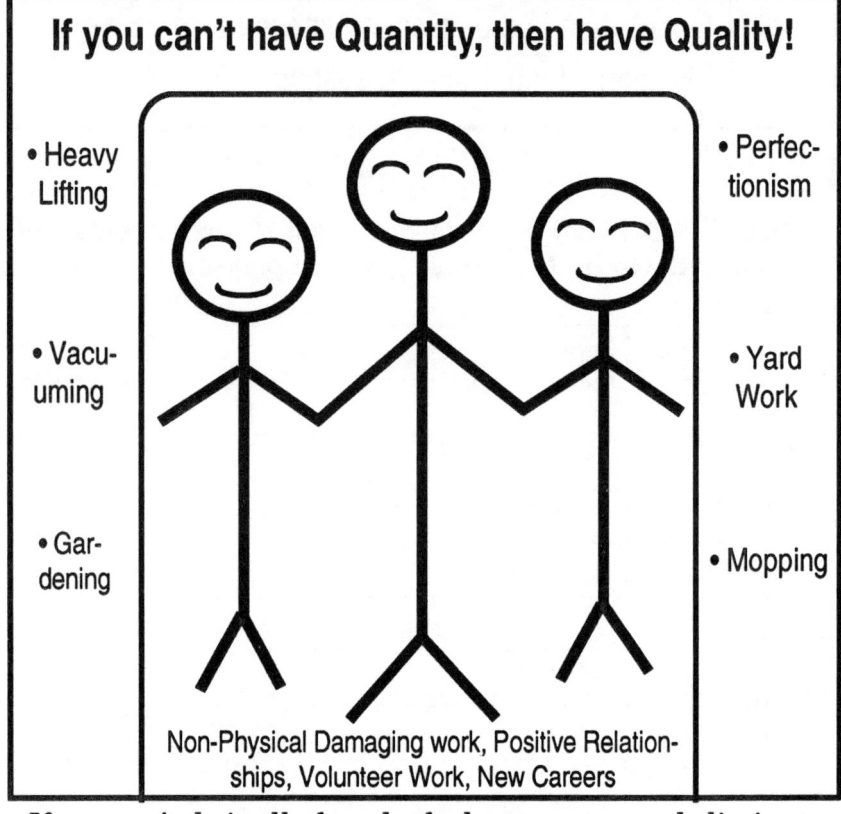

If you can't have Quantity, then have Quality!

- Heavy Lifting
- Vacuuming
- Gardening

- Perfectionism
- Yard Work
- Mopping

Non-Physical Damaging work, Positive Relationships, Volunteer Work, New Careers

If you can't do it all, then do the best you can and eliminate the unnecessary and injurious activities.

before or making time to focus on small pleasures, many people report that their sense of priorities shifts. As Mary told us: "Maybe it is not so important to keep the house clean or to do the yard work if it affects my health." Others report enjoying the sunsets and the flowers and the daily pleasures which they ignored before. Learning to value people and relationship helps them get in touch with aspects of themselves they hadn't before. When you have less energy and can't do it all, spend your energy on what is most important to you and delegate as much of the rest as possible. Take a few moments to make a list of what you like to do and prioritize from most to least important. Which activities can you *eliminate?* Which are most important to do?

_____

_____

_____

_____

_____

_____

_____

_____

_____

_____

Seeking Your Higher Self

How can we use our strengths to help us through the pain crisis? We have talked about different aspects of you that constitute your identity and asked you to look at those parts of yourself that rise above the physical sphere. We will call this part Self with a capital S, that part of you that has always been with you. The Self has been referred to as an inner or higher Self by some psychologists and an Inner Guide by others. Some may call it the "unconscious" or "the center". Regardless of how we refer to it, it is essentially that part of us that "has always been" and that is something larger than the daily physical being. This is the Self that is underneath all the "Who am I?" descriptions. It is the self-wisdom that comes to us in those moments when we feel connected to the present. That Self is the wise person within each one of us that can help us at different times in our lives. When we connect with that aspect of ourselves, we know what we need to do to transform the pain experience into a new meaningful life. We can use the Self to help us when we jump from one trapeze bar to another.

There are many ways of getting in touch with our inner Self to help us heal and to find meaning in spite of the pain. Dreams, deep states of meditation and moments when we feel truly connected with others are times when we can use our Self to help us in moments of crisis. If you have already learned to use meditation or other relaxation methods, you may attempt to visualize that higher Self and ask for its help in dealing with your pain.

Our higher Self goes beyond the physical. We have already seen how stress can affect us physically and intensify the pain. Stress occurs when we are disconnected from ourselves, from other people and from the world at large. We have so far explored separation and lack of connectedness on the *personal* level: what goes on in our minds and thoughts affects our bodies. We have also discussed pain and stress on an *interpersonal level:* when we isolate ourselves from others, it affects our physical well-being as well. We have seen how crucial social support is to health and healing. How we are connected to the world is the third level from which we experience pain. The *transpersonal or spiritual level* has to do with how connected we feel to our universe. How do I see the world and what is my relationship to it? This essentially addresses our search for meaning when life is difficult.

The Search for Meaning

When we are sick, we start questioning our basic belief systems about ourselves and our universe. How we see the world determines to a large extent how we can face the trauma of pain and survive those periods between trapeze bars. We have already talked about how feelings of helplessness and pessimism, and of being out of control, can affect our immune system and make us more vulnerable to pain. When we see the universe as hostile and ourselves as helpless victims, we feel doomed. It is when we are suffering that we get in touch with our basic beliefs about the world and start asking questions like "Why me?" or "What did I do to deserve this?" Most people have a theory about why they are ill, and that may determine to a large extent their response to their illness. For example, underneath Marion's professional exterior was the basic conviction that she was "bad", "one big wart" who was being punished for her sins.

There is a great deal of reinforcement for this type of thinking with all of the literature that tells us that we are responsible for our illness. Many people, unfortunately, misinterpret that to mean that they *caused* their pain and are to blame for it. It is when we get ill that we start looking at our basic views about the world we live in. Some people who have intellectually rejected any form of religion for most of their lives will start looking at their childhood religious beliefs which may come back to haunt them. Others will question their faith and ask "Is there a God?" "And if there is, why is this happening?"

The search for meaning in life—trying to make sense out of the pain—is very important. Viktor Frankl (1959), a psychiatrist who spent many years in one of the most horrible concentration camps during the second World War, addresses this question in his book *Man's Search for Meaning*. He writes that man's concern is not to gain pleasure or avoid pain but to see a meaning in his life and that man is ready to suffer if his suffering has a larger meaning. You will remember that one of the attitudes that was most important in keeping executives illness-resistant was that of commitment, having something important to believe in, having a purpose.

The question of suicide—whether life is worth living if it's so painful—ultimately has to do with one's beliefs about meaning in life. There are not many people who at some time or other don't contemplate suicide, as Lenny did, but knowing that he had kids to raise and a family that loved him gave significance to his life beyond the physical sphere. He had a purpose and an obligation.

The search for meaning is essential to our well-being and can exceed the physical aspects of pain. Erik Erikson, a leading psychoanalyst, has talked of the last stages of life where the crisis between trapeze bars has to do with ego integration versus despair. If one looks at one's life and feels it has had a purpose to it, one can feel integrated and ready to face death. Despair happens when one feels that life has been aimless. When people are in chronic pain, this looking inward and asking "Does my life have meaning?" comes earlier than the last stages of life.

Terry Anderson who was held hostage for a long time by terrorists states that we come closest to God in our worst moments. In times of crisis, it is important to address our spiritual beliefs. Whereas psychology has traditionally shied away from those subjects, there is increasing recognition that the spiritual needs have to be addressed in illness, as much as the physical and the emotional ones. The humanistic psychologist Abraham Maslow has discussed the need for us not only to find personal but spiritual meaning in our lives. As psychologists working with people in pain, we would be remiss if we didn't discuss this aspect in the book. However, it is beyond our professional expertise to provide counseling in this area except to encourage you to explore your spiritual views with a clergyman of your denomination.

In the space below, write down your basic beliefs about how you see your meaning in life. What questions do you have? How are these beliefs helping or hurting you?

_____

_____

_____

_____

_____

_____

_____

_____

_____

_____

Finding meaning and a purpose in life is essential to our well-being and can help us cope with pain. Cecil E. Maranville (1994) who has written on his living with chronic pain for many years states: "The strength of the spirit must be our focus, not the strength of the body."

Since many people find a mission in life through their work, being off work may make one feel useless. Many persons with chronic pain are unable to hold a regular job and may be receiving disability benefits. If you are not working, we very strongly encourage you to do volunteer work. When you volunteer, it brings out the best in you and gives you a purpose to get up in the morning. The advantage of volunteer work is you can do it on your terms—even only two hours a week—and if you can't make it to work at times, you don't have to go. People who have volunteered have reported that this has provided them ten times what they have put in. It boosts self-esteem and gives you the feeling of connectedness and sharing with others.

"To do something where you feel your life counts, to do something that makes a difference—it really makes me feel alive again. I never realized how much more this is giving me back than I am putting into it. *Volunteer work has given me my life back."* Dora is articulate in her feelings about being useful again. There are many volunteer activities that you can do and where you would be welcome: churches, schools, museums, favorite charities and organizations or hospitals.

No matter what your physical condition, you can make a difference in the world. Lisa, the woman with cancer who was bedridden, could still write letters to her congressman and feel useful. Illness or pain does not diminish your capacity for loving and caring and giving. Pain does not take away your identity. Your higher Self, the one that connects to others and to the world, goes beyond pain. As Bill summarized it: "We have all forgotten the basics—that's what it is: going back to the basics."

"Going back to the basics" can enable people with chronic pain to resolve the pain crisis and "get their life back", as Dora did. It is a new notion of acceptance which Cheri Register expresses very well: "from a preoccupation with illness to gratitude for all that is good in life to an unconditional love of life; I have also moved from sorrow and fear to a glossy-surfaced contentment to a true joy in living." She goes on to state: "I can even affirm my illness—a very private, personal suffering—as my own share in life's condition: not an aberration, not deviant, simply a way of life." (p.275)

Summary

How can we learn to find meaning in life in spite of the pain? Rather than comparing our life now with how it used to be, we can see it as a different life and try to find meaning within its parameters. Acceptance is not only finding meaning in living in spite of the pain but working at ways to transform the energy of the suffering into something worthwhile. Health is not just the absence of illness but also adding positive experiences to our lives . If you can't have quantity, focus on quality. We need to focus on our higher Self that goes beyond physical boundaries. We must address our pain crisis on a personal, interpersonal and transpersonal level and explore our spiritual beliefs to find a direction in life through volunteer work and other activities. We must learn to get back to basics.

Chapter 10

Recap, Relapse, Readings & Resources

We have seen how pain affects all areas of functioning and walked you through the stages of loss on your way to getting off the pain roller coaster and getting on with your life. If you have been diligently working on this program and have come this far, this may be a good time to look back and re-assess your gains. The following questions may help you along.

Recap

Go back to Chapter 1 and review your goals. What changes have you made so far?

_____

_____

_____

_____

_____

_____

_____

What do you still need to work on?

_____

_____

_____

_____

_____

_____

Go back to Chapter 2 and review how we experience pain. What can you still do to intercept pain at the signal level?

_____

_____

_____

_____

_____

_____

_____

_____

At the message level?

_____

_____

_____

_____

_____

_____

_____

At the response level?

_____

_____

_____

_____

_____

_____

_____

Review the questions in Chapter 3 and see if you need to make any more changes in your communication with your health providers to make them partners instead of adversaries.

_____

_____

_____

_____

_____

_____

_____

_____

_____

_____

Reread Chapter 4 as it is the most important chapter in the book. Are you controlling your pain or are you allowing it to control you? Are you pacing yourself adequately? What do you still need to do to gain more control?

_____

_____

_____

_____

_____

_____

_____

_____

_____

_____

Review Chapter 5 and ask yourself: Am I allowing negative emotions and stress to close the pain gate? What do I still need to do to reduce the stress? What are some ways of increasing pleasure in my life to bring out the brain's natural pain killers?

_____

_____

_____

_____

_____

_____

_____

_____

_____

_____

Go back to Chapter 6 and ask yourself: Are there any pain behaviors to eliminate? What about pain talk? Have I stopped using pain talk that only makes me hurt more? Have I educated my family and friends about pain talk? Have I substituted humor and laughter in my life instead?

_____

_____

_____

_____

_____

_____

_____

_____

_____

_____

Review Chapter 7 and ask yourself: Am I starting to use my mind as an ally to lower the pain? Am I using some form of relaxation method four times daily? Have I been successful at changing the way I think about pain?

_____

_____

_____

_____

_____

_____

_____

_____

_____

Reread Chapter 8 and ask: Am I communicating more openly with my family? Have I discussed sexuality with my partner? What do I still need to do to open up communication? What about other people? Do I need to decrease isolation?

_____

_____

_____

_____

_____

_____

_____

_____

_____

Review the exercises in Chapter 9. What can you still do to find meaning in life in spite of the pain?

_____

_____

_____

_____

_____

_____

_____

_____

_____

_____

We hope you continue to look at this workbook and your responses from time to time. Dealing with pain is a daily event, just as dealing with life is a daily undertaking. Even if you have made significant changes by now, you will still want to reread portions of the book.

Relapse

Although you may have met many of your goals by now and have learned to lower your pain and go on with your life, you may still have setbacks from time to time. Relapse is not an unanticipated event—it is *expected*. When that happens, don't fear it. Don't tell yourself, "What's the use? Nothing helps." Just remember that temporary relapses or setbacks are part of all learning and change, and expect to experience them in those spaces between trapeze bars. When you have a setback and feel like you are back to square one, see it as a *cue* to go back and reread the book. View it as a signal to practice the new skills you have learned. When your pain comes back, ask yourself: What is my body telling me? And what do I need to do to take care of myself right now? Do I need to pace myself? Do I need to relax? Should I work on my thinking patterns?

As we said at the beginning of this book, this workbook is

not to be used in lieu of a pain program. We would like to list here some of the major pain organizations that you can contact to get referrals and resources. In addition, we want to suggest some other books that you may wish to read that can serve as resources for areas that were not covered in detail in this book.

Readings

The following books are also recommended that provide valuable information on chronic pain:

Vasudevan, S.D. (1993). *Pain: A Four-Letter Word You Can Live With*. Milwaukee, WI: Montgomery Media, Inc. (Brief, clear, well-written book that gives a summary of pain, pain management and treatment).

Bresler, D.E. and Trubo, R. (1979). *Freeing Yourself from Pain*. New York: Simon & Schuster. (Detailed, comprehensive book on pain and pain treatment).

Mellwain, H.M., Fulghum, B., Silverfield, J., Burnette, M.C., & Germain, B.F. (1994). *Winning with Chronic Pain*. Amherst, NY: Prometheus Books. (Discusses treatment plans for different types of pain).

Root, L. Y Kiernan, T. (1973). *Oh, My Aching Back*. N.Y.: Signet. (Excellent book on back pain).

Borysenko, J. (1987). *Minding the Body, Mending the Mind*. New York: Bantam. (Reviews the mind's effect on healing).

Resources

American Chronic Pain Association
P.O. Box 850
Rocklin, CA 95677]
(916) 632-0922

National Chronic Pain Outreach Association, Inc.
7979 Old Georgetown Rd., Ste. 100
Bethesda, MD 20814-2429
(301) 652-4948

American Pain Society
Skokie, IL
(708) 965-2776

International Association for the Study of Pain
909 NE 43rd St., Ste.306
Seattle, WA 98105
(206) 547-2157

American Academy of Pain Medicine (AAPM)
5700 Old Orchard Road
Skokie, IL 60077
(708) 966-9510

References

Brand, P. & Yancey. (1988). *Pain: The Gift Nobody Wants.* New York: Harper Collins.

Cousins, N. (1976). Anatomy of an illness. *New England Journal of Medicine,* 295, 1457-62.

Frankl, V.E. (1959). *Man's Search for Meaning.* New York: Washington Square Press.

Kobasa, S.C. (1979). Stressful life events, personality, and health: An inquiry into hardiness. *Journal of Personality and Social Psychology,* 37, 1-11.

Kobasa, S.C. (1984). How much stress can you survive? *American Health Magazine.* September, 64-77.

Kubler-Ross, E. (1969). *On Death and Dying.* New York: McMillan.

Maranville, C.E. (1994). Dealing with disability, yours and your neighbor's. Unpublished manuscript. (Reprints available by writing to C.E. Maranville, 3033 E. Cortez St., Phoenix, AZ 85028-1921.)

Melzach, R. & Wall, P.D. (1965). Pain mechanisms: A new theory. *Science,* 150, 971-79.

Ornstein, R.E. & Sobel, D.S. (1989) *Healthy Pleasures.* Reading, MA: Addison-Wesley.

Potkay, C.R. & Allen, B.P. (1986). Personality: Theory, Research and Applications. Monterey, CA: Brooks/Cole.

Register, C. (1987). *Living with Chronic Illness.* New York: Free Press.

Root, L. & Kiernan, T. (1973). *Oh, My Aching Back.* New York: Signet.

Sarton, M. (1980). The country of pain. *Halfway to Silence.* New York: Norton.

Shealy, C.N. (1976). *The Pain Game.* Millbrae, CA: Celestial Arts.

Siegel, B. (1987). *Love, Medicine and Miracles.* San Francisco: Harper & Rowe.

Westberg, G. (1962). *A Short Book on The Process of Grieving.* Fortress Press.

About the Authors

Barry W. Weiss, Ph.D. is a psychologist in private practice who has worked with pain patients for many years and specializes in the treatment of chronic pain. He is the former program director of St. Luke's Pain and Stress Center in Phoenix, Arizona. Lillie Weiss, Ph.D. is a psychologist in private practice, Adjunct Associate Professor at Arizona State University, Department of Psychology and the author of several books on psychology.

GETTING OFF THE PAIN ROLLER COASTER

Psychological Aspects of Pain and Pain Management

by

Barry W. Weiss, Ph.D.

Lillie Weiss, Ph.D.

This book is a detailed step-by-step guide for persons with chronic pain, as well as their families, their loved ones and all those who treat and represent them. Written in a clear, conversational style in workbook format, it combines sound psychological principles with practical tools to lower pain, reduce the frustrations associated with living in chronic pain and live a happier life. It can be used by persons with chronic pain and adopted by therapists and health care providers in pain centers.

—— ORDER FORM ——

Please complete all information and mail to:

Golden Psych Press
4202 N. 32nd St. #H
Phoenix, AZ 85018
(602) 954-6998

Please send _____ copy(ies) of *Getting Off the Pain Roller Coaster: Psychological Aspects of Pain and Pain Management* @ $14.95 each.

Sub Total _____

Postage and Handling __$2.00___

Total _____

☐ Check enclosed   ☐ Money Order enclosed

Ship to:

Name _____

Address _____

City/State/Zip _____